Throw Your Heart Over

Book Three • Stonegate Series

Tudor Robins

Tudor Robins
www.tudorrobins.ca

Publisher's Note: This is a work of fiction. Names, characters, places, and incidents are a product of the author's imagination. Locales and public names are sometimes used for atmospheric purposes. Any resemblance to actual people, living or dead, or to businesses, companies, events, institutions, or locales is completely coincidental.

Book Layout © 2017 BookDesignTemplates.com

Throw Your Heart Over / Tudor Robins. -- 1st ed.
ISBN 978-1-9991338-0-1

Other Books by Tudor Robins:

Island Series:
Six-Month Horse (Prequel)
Appaloosa Summer (Book One)
Wednesday Riders (Book Two)
Join Up (Book Three)
Faults (Book Four)

Stonegate Series:
Objects in Mirror (Book One)
After Lucas (Book Two)

Chris & Tilly Series:
Meant to Be

Chapter One

The alarm goes while I'm still in the shower.

Late! Late! Late! I hate running late.

My anxiety level ratchets up as the chime drones on relentlessly.

Dee-dee-dah ...

I slam off the water.

Dee-dee-dah ...

Grope for a towel.

Dee-dee-dah ...

Set a soaking wet foot on the bathroom tile and lurch as it goes out from under me. Balance myself on the counter top, yank open the drawer – releasing a much louder *dee-dee-dah* – and smack the snooze button.

I turn back toward the bathmat and catch a glimpse of myself in the unfogged part of the mirror.

And that's when I remember.

I'm not going to be late.

I lean in, turn my chin left, then right. Lift it and peer underneath. All clear. Not a blemish in sight.

No more staring and agonizing.

No telling myself I'll pop "just one" whitehead – just the very worst one. Followed by just one more, then just one more.

No sudden realization that just one has turned into my whole face. That it looks worse than when I started.

No freaking out when the alarm goes off for the second time, reminding me I should have been out of the bathroom two minutes ago; knowing I can never, ever face the world with my face as swollen and red as it is.

That's all behind me.

All I have to do this morning is finish drying the parts of me that haven't already air-dried, slap some light, high-UV moisturizer on my face, skim on some lip balm and, maybe, a bit of mascara, and I can go to my room, pull on my clothes and leave for school with time to spare.

I'm fully dressed, slinging my backpack over my shoulder when I hear it again – *dee-dee-dah* – the alarm coming out of snooze mode.

I cross the hall to the bathroom, lever the protective battery panel off with my fingernail, and pop the batteries out. *There. Done. No more.*

I should throw them out.

I look at the garbage can tucked in the corner by the sink ... and hesitate.

Drop the separated clock and batteries back into my drawer.

I'll probably never need them again. Hopefully. Fingers crossed.

And now, if I don't go, I *will* be late.

***

Jostle, push, joggle. Mumbled, *"I'm sorry*'s and *"Excuse me*'s.

A girl to my left, phone jammed to her ear, "... I know – can you believe it? That's exactly what I told him ..."

A guy taking his life in his hands by dropping to a knee to tie his shoelace. *You're going to get run over ...* I think.

It's early days yet, and I'm still ninety parts overwhelmed, ten parts energized by the sea of humanity that surges from an otherwise quiet campus at each change of class, but I've learned how to deal with it; get in the right stream and let it carry me along.

Straight ahead are the doors leading into the building containing my next class. A complete bottleneck, but it will work out; it always does, somehow.

We'll all get in, and the crowd will immediately thin, with some heading up, others down. Some peeling into the common area, and others taking the covered passage to the Athletic Centre.

My mind wanders to Em, at her school two hundred kilometres away, and over a hundred years older than mine. I've been on her classic grey stone campus and I can't imagine it ever teeming with students like this.

Calm, polite, sedate, are the words that come to mind when I think of that place.

Also, *not for me.*

I've climbed one floor now, and am faced with an expanse of floor-to-ceiling windows. As has become my habit, I hunt out a spot that will throw my own reflection back at me.

I glance around to make sure nobody's watching. I'm extra careful ever since two of my sisters – over for Sunday dinner – stumbled across me peering into the mirror in our front hall. "Glad you love your reflection so much, Ellie." "Never met a mirror you didn't like."

Which of course, is not it at all. Quite the opposite. I'm double-checking. Making sure I still look OK. That I can face new people. Ensuring nobody's going to be staring at a spot high on my cheek while they talk to me – distracted from eye contact by the latest eruption of my acne.

A shaft of sunlight falls across the smooth skin of my cheeks and forehead, and my eyes re-adjust to take in the view of buildings that are brutalist, and modernist, and just-plain brand new.

Some people have been known to call them ugly, but this place suits me.

It suited me even more once I found out I was being offered an entrance scholarship.

Also, there was Dr. Hamilton. How could I move away from the safe haven of her quiet office, the relief of her kind bluntness – "The fact is, you have severe, scarring acne. The good news is, I can help" – and the results she'd given me?

Even if our family could afford for me to leave town for university, I might not find another Dr. Hamilton in a strange city.

After a final glance in the glass, I turn away, climb the second flight of stairs, and push through the double doors into the corridor only to find the room numbers inexplicably start with four, instead of two.

OK, time to hunt down my class.

***

When I finally find the classroom, up another funny half-flight of stairs and around a corner, there's only one empty table left.

All the others have at least one person sitting at them, and a few are already full with two occupants. From the way they're chatting, I assume those are people who already know each other.

I don't know anyone. Which is fine. This early in the year, I didn't expect to. With the exception of my full-on friendship with Em, I've always been pretty good at keeping myself to myself. I cross the room and take one of the seats at the last vacant table.

Once I've sat down, a girl comes in and drops into the empty seat closest to the door.

A guy comes in, catches sight of another guy, and we all listen to "Bro!" and "Dude!" and "It's ya' boy!" as what appears to be a high school reunion takes place.

Then a girl steps into the doorway. She scans the room and, for a minute, I think one of my high school classmates is here after all. Then I realize I don't actually know her. I do recognize her – that's true enough. Even though I've only been on campus a few days, there are a few people I keep crossing paths with, and she's one of them. I've passed her coming out of the bathroom while I was on my way in. Stood in line behind her at the vending machines. Saw her on one side of the quad while I was walking on the other.

She has glasses that scream librarian, and she must have a closet full of overalls because that's all I've ever seen her wear.

I've noticed her because she's that bit different from all the other late-teen-to-early-twenty-somethings roaming around campus wearing the same brand of shoes, and jeans, and lots and lots of identical backpacks (hers is a vintage camping backpack absolutely covered in badges and patches).

I've also noticed her because her skin looks just the way mine used to – the way I keep thinking mine does –

but where I spent the better part of a year wearing turtle-necks whenever the weather would reasonably let me get away with it, and letting my hair fall forward across my cheeks, she wears her curly hair back; wrestled into two bumpy braids.

Without having ever met her, I'm in awe of this brave person.

Now, her eyes connect with mine, and they crinkle at the corners, and a smile spreads across her face – and I remember, this is another thing I've been noticing about her; how her face is always wide-open with happiness – and she heads straight across the room to my table.

I've spent a long time trying hard to not be stand-out, or noticeable; wanting nothing more than to fade into the background. For the last chunk of my life just blend-ing in has been my main aim.

But she's dropping into the seat next to mine and say-ing, "Hey!" and it's the 'hey' of old friends and long-time-no-see, and I wonder if she's confused me with somebody else, but just then the professor comes in, so all I can do is shoot her a quick smile back, before opening my book and picking up my pen.

***

Our prof is mid-stream in a complex explanation when the clock ticks to 4:25. There may not be bells, or chimes, like in high school, but there are shuffling books, sliding chairs, coughs.

"OK, OK," the professor runs a hand through his hair. "So I'm not riveting enough for you to want to stay late."

The girl next to me speaks up. "It's not that. It's that the American Sign Language class is waiting to come in." She points at the door.

The prof grins at her. "Of course that's it. That makes so much more sense."

How does she do it? How does she know just what to say, and how to say it? How does she have the guts to speak up when she knows the whole class will turn and look at her?

She taps my wrist with one of my pens that escaped earlier in the class, rolling over to her side of the table. I reach for it and she holds out her hand. "Addy." Then before I can say anything she adds, "I can't believe it's you."

"It's me?"

"Yes! The pretty girl I keep noticing everywhere. I've wondered who you are, then I walk into Legal Studies and ... *voila*."

She noticed me? "I've noticed you, too."

"I wanted to meet you," she says.

Because it's one of those statements that feels rude not to respond to – like "I love you / I love you, too" – I say, "I wanted to meet you, too."

She rises to her feet. "Well, I told you I'm Addy, so ..."

"I ... oh ..." Could it be just this easy? How did I make friends with Em? I can't really remember, and for quite a while I haven't really been in "making new friends" mode. But now ... maybe? I mean, why not? "I'm Ellie."

"Well, Ellie, where are you heading?"

***

She walks me to the long, covered area outside the Athletic Centre chock-a-block with bikes of all sizes, shapes, colours, and price points. "Mine's over there." I point.

"Oh, wow. I'm impressed."

I shrug. "It's not that far of a bike ride, and it's mostly on paths."

"It's not the bike ride," she says. "Although, don't get me wrong – that does impress me – but I have no idea how you find your bike out of all these hundreds and hundreds of other bikes."

I tilt my head. "Is it possible you're maybe not exactly a bike person?"

She laughs, head back, showing bright white teeth. "I am in no way a bike person!"

"Well, this is mine." The lowering rays of the sun are slanted under the roof across my cross-bar and I lay my hand on the sun-warmed frame. It's purple, scratched, the underside is coated with road grime, and the newest thing on the bike is the sticker proclaiming **One Less Car** wrapped around the seat tube.

"Is there a reason you have three locks on it?"

"Um, well, I like this bike."

It's the understatement of the year. I adore this inanimate object with a depth and ferocity I know is completely irrational. It's just done so much for me, though. Taken me everywhere I want to go. Never let me down. Sometimes I talk to it.

OK – honesty – I talk to it more than I talk to most people.

Which makes it a miracle I'm standing here with Addy. Who's now reaching out, saying, "Hand me your phone. While you're unlocking Fort Knox there, I'll enter myself in your contacts."

By the time I have the locks removed and stowed she's holding the phone back for me.

I take it. Read **Adeline Murphy**. I flick my eyes from the screen to her face. "It's a really pretty name."

"Hmm ..." She doesn't drop my gaze. "Too bad I'm not."

"What?" My heart hammers, while guilt that I've messed up floods me. I was sure I was maintaining eye contact. Positive I wasn't staring at the angry cyst stretched over her left cheekbone.

And I *do* think she's pretty. Actually, she's better than pretty – she's captivating. That smile, her sparkly eyes, the way she puts herself out there. You just want to be near her. Even I want to be near her, and I rarely want to be near anyone who isn't Em, or my family. Often enough I don't even want to be near my sisters.

But I know better to say that. Better than to repeat some of the well-meaning things I heard in the lead-up to finally, finally seeing Dr. Hamilton:

- *"You have a very pretty smile."* Usually followed by. *"If you just use that smile, nobody will ever notice your skin."*
- Or the closely related, *"No one else thinks it's nearly as bad as you do."*
- Then there's the less-than-helpful, *"Have you ever tried (insert miracle cure)?"*
- And, the always-brilliant kicker – *"Beauty is only skin deep"* – which, yeah, my *skin* is exactly what we're talking about here – remember?

Although, I'm suddenly feeling a little more forgiving of those people, because really, what am I supposed to say?

I stare her in the eyes, while finally coming to a full and complete understanding of the meaning of "deer caught in headlights" and she wrinkles her nose.

"It's OK," she says. "Thanks for looking me in the eye, instead of staring at my latest and worst zit and, also, thanks for not recommending that I eat less chocolate."

I admire Addy for being brave. This is a moment to be brave. I use up all my breath and still end up managing not-much-better than a whisper. "I get it."

"Pardon me?"

"I'm on my last month of Acnegon."

"Oh," she says. "Wow. It's ... so, it really works?"

I dodge another awkward moment by channeling my sisters, who live by the axiom that sarcasm is always an acceptable stand-in for seriousness. "Well, obviously. I'm only killing time here while my agent negotiates my international modeling contract."

I'm still wondering, *Was that not appropriate? Was it too flip?* When we both turn at the sound of, "Addy! Addy-Addy-Addy!" Three girls, arms linked, come around the corner of the bike shelter. "We're starving! Are you coming to the caf with us?"

"Some of my floormates," she tells me. "I live in res."

"Oh," I say. "Cool. I've never seen inside a residence."

"It's not all it's cracked up to be," she says.

So, yeah, maybe too flip. She doesn't want to encourage me.

She points to my phone. "You have my number now. If you're ever staying late on campus, text me. We can grab food together and study in my room." She winks. "You might as well experience the wonders of residence before your modeling career takes off and you get used to five-star hotels."

Chapter Two

Me: So, you were right …

    Em: **About what? I mean, of course I was, but about what, specifically?**

Me: **Let's just say I'm at Stationary Stationery.**

Em: **Ha! Told you!**

Me: **Is that your version of sympathy?**

Em again: **No, that's me gloating. I told you not to buy any school stuff before classes started. I said you'd only have to go back after the first week. How long is your list?**

Me: **Long enough. You must have to buy stuff too?**

Em: **Loose-leaf can wait. I'm about to get on a bus for a rock-climbing team-building activity with everyone from my floor in residence.**

Me: **Well, thank goodness I'm at Stationary Stationery, 'cause yours sounds like it'll suck.**

Em: **It's going to suck rocks (get it…?)**

Me: **Have fun. Gotta go. There's a pack of loose-leaf calling my name.**

They sell patterned loose-leaf.

I had no idea.

It's got decorative borders around the margins. There are three patterns to choose from. Purplish paisley, pink flowers, or blue stars. It's surprisingly pretty. It's also surprisingly expensive.

I snap a picture of the purple paisley paper and text it to Em: **Decorative loose-leaf. Discuss.**

I'm thinking nobody needs ornamental loose-leaf while, for some reason, still staring at it, when I take a step that bumps me into another body.

"Ellie?"

I whirl around. "Oh! Hi!" It's automatic polite instinct. Say hi first, figure out who it is later. Except ... I hold the smile on my face while my brain races. She is so, so familiar. Pretty. Really pretty. Older than me – than any of my friends – but younger than any of our parents. Who *is* she?

I turn back to the newcomer. "It's Laney," she says. "Em's riding coach?"

Of course. In my mind she belongs in the wide-open outdoors, wearing dusty boots and faded jeans with effortless style, walking casually and confidently around the big animals I love watching, but am quite scared of.

"Yes," I say. "Sorry. I didn't recognize you here."

She wrinkles her nose. "I know – I do most of my shopping at tack stores. But I was visiting a friend who lives nearby and I ran out of staples the other day." She laughs. "Staples! One day you have a box of a thousand, and then they're gone ... anyway, sorry, completely irrelevant – how are you?"

"I'm, yeah, I'm good. I mean, I made it through my first classes so, you know – new stuff to get used to ..."

Stop talking, I think. Then amend it to, *Stop babbling*. Laney though, since she's kind, is nodding as though I'm making perfect sense. "For Em, too, I guess. Lucas is really going to miss her."

Lucas. He's not that far away from her. Same city, even if different campuses. They'll still see each other several times a week. Then I realize Laney, of course, means the horse Lucas. The animal with the long tail, and the exquisitely adorable ears, who Em assures me wouldn't hurt a fly, but who has a body so enormous, and hooves so hard, that he might hurt much more than a fly without ever meaning to.

Now I'd almost welcome back the babbling version of me because I have no idea how to respond. What do you say when somebody tells you a horse is going to miss a person? Do horses miss people?

I stare at Laney hoping she'll rescue me again, and she does; putting her hand on my upper arm, and squeezing. "Oh …" she says. "Of course. I'm so insensitive. You'll miss Em too. But you'll be tied up with classes. And didn't Em tell me you're a great ringette player? That will keep you busy."

At least I can speak on this topic. "I aged out of ringette. My club doesn't have a U19 team this year." It's true there's a university team, but although I was a solid ringette player, I wasn't brilliant. Definitely not university-level, so as much as it's strange not to be heading back to the rink with my teammates from years and years of playing, ringette is done for me. For now, anyway.

I think of explaining all that to Laney, then think better of it. If horses don't mean much to me, ringette probably means less to her. I shake my head. "Anyway, short story: no ringette. Which is why I'm here, shopping for school supplies, instead of skating in a rink in the boonies somewhere." The laugh I force out sounds fake even to me.

Laney's eyes light up. "I know!"

I blink, twice. "You know … what?"

"I know the perfect thing you could do!" She grins. "Are you going to the check-out? Walk with me, and I'll tell you."

I fall into step beside her. "Tell me what?"

"You could join my Learn to Ride program!"

"I ..." *Don't laugh. Don't yelp. She's trying to be nice.* "I mean, that would be great if I wasn't terrified of horses."

"Pshaw! Lucas is a gentle giant. I'm sure Em would love it if you used him. It would make her feel better about being away."

"Did you just say, 'Pshaw?'"

She flicks her eyes away from the items she's unloading onto the counter and back to me. "Are you changing the subject?"

"Yes. I'm trying to gloss over the 'giant' part of the 'gentle giant.' That's what worries me."

The check-out girl tells her the total, and Laney digs in her bag without breaking off our conversation. "Listen, Ellie. Horses have helped more than one person through a transition, or a hard time, or whatever you want to call it. You don't have to look any farther than Em to see that. I know you can do it, or I wouldn't even suggest it. So think about it, and if you decide to give it a try, I'll help you, and you'll do great."

What am I even supposed to say to her? It doesn't really matter. She's leaving and I'll probably never see her again, so I settle on, "Sure. OK. I'll think about it."

She picks up her shopping bag. "If you want more information, the program's listed on the Stonegate website – just Google it – I'm running the program in conjunction with them." A phone pings from somewhere on her person and she says, "Oh, I've got to go! Listen, there's one spot left in the class. We'd love to have you there."

And she's gone.

"That'll be six-ninety-seven."

"Pardon me?"

The girl behind the counter is pointing at her display. "Six-ninety-seven. For the paper."

"Oh," I say. "Yeah. For the paper." I count out the money, and she hands me the paper and as I walk out of the store my phone pings.

Em: **What kind of person buys decorative loose-leaf?**

Me: **Um, yeah. About that ...**

***

Later, as I'm hole punching my new loose-leaf – because apparently, yes, you can pay six dollars and ninety-seven cents for loose-leaf and still have to punch your own holes in it – my phone rings.

I grab it, jam it under my shoulder, nearly drop it, and gasp out, "Yuh-huh?"

"Well, that's an awesome greeting!"

"Em! I didn't even check the display first. I'm so excited it's you."

"Well we said we'd stay in touch – and not just by text – although I have to warn you, Lucas is going to be here in a second, and before you give me a hard time; it's the first time I've seen him all week, but I had to know how it's going for you, so spill!"

"Good. I found all my classes ... eventually. And, you'll never guess who I saw today right after you and I texted."

"Who?"

"Laney."

"Laney? Like riding Laney? In the city. That's so weird ..."

I snort. "No, what's weird is she wants me to ride."

"Ride?" The uplift in Em's voice sets off internal alarm bells. Should. Not. Have. Mentioned. That.

"Oh, just some Learn to Ride program. It's completely not possible. You know, money, and time, and me being shit-scared of horses. So, are you and Lucas going out for dinner?"

"Nuh-uh. No way. You're not skipping past Learn to Ride Ellie-bellie. You should do it."

"Of course you think I should do it."

"Of course I do, because it's such a great idea that I'm embarrassed I didn't think of it. Also ..." She smothers the sparkle out of her voice. "... I miss him, you know. It was really hard to leave Lucas behind at the barn. If I knew you were going out to see him every week – well – it would be a load off my mind." I half-expect her to throw in a sniff at the end.

"I know what you're doing."

Now she does sniff. Twice. Then she bursts into laughter. "OK, OK. You can't blame me for trying. Is it working?"

"What do you think?"

"I think I'm very persuasive."

In the background I hear noises and scuffling, followed by Lucas's familiar voice yelling. "Hey Ellie – if she's trying to persuade you to do something, you know you might as well just give in and do it."

I yell back. "Thanks for the advice, Lucas!"

Em's voice comes through loud and clear. "So what do you think?"

"I think you'd better go out for dinner."

"Happy riding!" she sing-songs.

"Em! I'm not ..." But she's already gone.

And I'm looking at the calendar hung over my desk – the one Em gave me for my birthday topped with a collage of pictures, including one of her grinning on Lucas's back – and I'm noticing all the empty squares that would normally be jammed with ringette practices.

Chapter Three

Sunday morning when I come awake, the sun's up, but it's not really morning. Not by any normal person's measure.

Especially not on a weekend – later on there will be a line-up for the brunch place in the village, and the sidewalks will be thronged with people dropping into coffee shops, and patios, and walking their dogs. This early, though, all normal people – especially just-starting-university teenagers – are supposed to be snoring in the hazy post dawn light filtering through closed curtains.

My brain's too busy to sleep though, so I pull on light running shorts and a form-fitting tank, and I run.

On my way to the end of my street, I make a mental list. Things to think about. The topic for my first short essay for English class. Survival strategies for my oldest sister's upcoming wedding. Whether I should pay for a professional tune-up for my bike, or just spend some time this afternoon doing as much maintenance as I know how to. And, because I know Em will ask me again, riding.

While I weave through the neighbourhood on my way to the paths that hug the shore of the river, I begin to work all these things through.

I've just started in on my essay topic when I pass my old high school. A couple of guys I recognize are shooting hoops on the outdoor court.

Friends of Rory's.

I cross to the far sidewalk.

Rory's gone. With Em away at university, and his parents posted out of town for a year for his dad's work, Rory's attending a residential sports school. I'm sure he's happy there.

I glance over, then quickly away.

The reason "I'm sure" Rory's happy, as opposed to knowing it firsthand, is that we don't talk anymore.

I keep my eyes fixed straight ahead, listen to the thwacking of the ball. If they keep dribbling, and shooting, it means they're not staring at me.

There's no nice way to say it. Rory dumped me when my skin went haywire.

I mean, I get it. Or, at least that's what I told Em when she clenched her fists and said, "I'm going to rip him to shreds."

I'd tried to be rational – mostly because it was logistically impossible for my best friend to never speak to her brother again, so I didn't want to put her in that position.

I'd said, "I've changed, Em. Not just my face ..." although, at the time, my face had felt like it was full of ball bearings that were on fire. "... I don't like going out anymore. And, at the risk of TMI, it's not like I really feel like kissing anyone right now."

"No, Ellie." Em had shaken her head. "You're still you. Just because whatever happened – hormones, or something else; something you can't control – that doesn't make you *not* Ellie. People who love you have to keep loving you."

That's the part that had made me sad – made the tears roll down my ravaged cheeks – because we both knew what she'd really just said. Rory clearly didn't love me. Not enough.

I keep running, focusing on bringing my breathing back to a steady rhythm I can maintain through my run.

Rory might have broken my heart, but he wasn't cruel. I'm sure he never said anything about me – my acne – to his friends.

Still, my steps come more smoothly and my heart rate settles once I've left the basketball court and its occupiers well behind me.

I hit the river paths and pass the flat rocks, covered with Inukshuks.

OK, back to my essay. I'm going to write about the unreliable narrator in poetry. *That was easy.*

I negotiate the banking curve skirting the river at its most dangerous point – where tiny, bird-bestrewn islands nestle so close to the shore people often try to swim to them, only to discover the currents are swift, strong, and swirling, and the bottom vanishes quickly from underfoot.

Wedding. The term "grin and bear it" was designed to get me through my role in my sister's wedding party. Bonus of grinning and bearing it is I guess I'll always be smiling in the photos which, since I generally dread having my photo taken, will at least make me look happy.

I run behind the War Museum and alongside the shuttered mills, and log weirs and dams. Behind the National Archives, the Parliament buildings, then climb the steep trail beside the tumble of locks spilling canal water – and boats – into the river.

Bike. I'm pretty handy with a wrench and I have an old t-shirt I can rip up for rags. Clean my bike as best I can now – pay for a complete tune-up before I put it away for the winter.

I turn back and one of the many vistas that make my city special is spread in front of me – treed hillside, blue sky, wide river, all in the shadow of the Peace Tower – and I have it entirely to myself.

Riding. I've already solved three out of four problems on this run. I'm going to empty my mind as I fly home and I can come back to riding later.

It's a long, long run and, by the time I'm done, everything I'm wearing is soaked through, and I have a raw spot where the seam of my tank top has rubbed the tender fish-belly white skin on the inside of my arm to a sore pink, and I really, desperately need a shower.

My parents are drinking coffee on the back deck in their pyjamas and it's not even nine a.m. and running has worked its usual magic. My body's tired, brain awake, and I'm ready to tackle my poetry essay.

As for riding, I'm finding it's a nice thing to keep tucked in the back of my mind. As long as I don't decide I'm definitely *not* doing it, the possibility remains that I *might*.

It's been hard for me to believe that things are changing. That this new, clear skin is *mine*, and that it will stay clear. That I can go out in the world and not have people stare at me. That, maybe, I could have the relationship I never quite got to enjoy with Rory.

But this riding thought ... well, it makes me feel like there *could* be some adventure in my life. Maybe.

In the meantime, though, I'd better get inside and wash this sweat off my face because the last thing I want is to have a break-out and know it was my own fault.

Chapter Four

I slide into my seat just as my dad places a platter of barbecued steaks in the middle of the table. My rail-thin, sweet-and-dainty looking sisters nearly knock over the jug of ice water in their rush to each snag the biggest steak while I, happy to have no competition, reach for the black bean and corn salad.

Melinda – the oldest, and most perfect, of my older, perfect sisters – takes her first bite, chews appreciatively, says, "Very good, Dad," then points her fork at me. "You were late."

I had Legal Studies again today, and Addy walked me to my bike again. We'd stood talking until the sun got so low it was shining right in my eyes. "Whoa!" I'd told her. "I'm supposed to be sitting at the dinner table in half-an-hour."

I pedaled hard and, even if the back of my t-shirt is still wet with sweat where my backpack covered it, I'm on time ... I think. "Late for what?"

"For choosing bridesmaid's dresses from the catalogue," Rachel says. "I dibsed spaghetti straps."

I'm still trying to catch up to the conversation, and, as usual it's Paige – the sister who lived at home with me the longest – who takes pity on me. She slides a brochure in my direction.

None of the bridesmaid's dresses it displays are pretty. The one with spaghetti straps, though, is definitely the least fluffy, frou-frou – whatever you want to call it – of the three. The one with cap sleeves is only marginally worse. Rachel gestures to it with her fork. "Paige is having that one."

Which means I'm in the high-necked, puffed sleeves, Cinderella-type version.

"It's OK," Paige speaks up. "I'll take the ugly dress."

Melinda's shoulders hike and she sets her steak-laden fork on the edge of her plate. "Excuse me? *Ugly?*"

"Come on, Melinda," Rachel says. "These aren't the world's prettiest dresses."

"Remind me – who's the bride?" Melinda asks.

"You are."

"So, who gets the world's prettiest dress?"

"Still," Paige says. "The one Ellie's supposed to wear is quite ... frumpy. Why can't we all have the strappy one?"

"Feel free to have a tacky matchy-matchy wedding when it's your turn," Melinda says. "My wedding is going to be classier than that."

Paige's eyes flick to the table. She was, indeed, very close to having her own wedding, until her forever-boyfriend decided they both needed to "experience more of the world," which, we later found out, meant he'd gotten somebody else pregnant.

Despite our sisterly support – "He'll experience the world of colic," "He'll experience the romance of living in a sleep-deprived relationship with a woman who probably never wants him to touch her again," – it took Paige a long time to smile again. Now she has a new boyfriend, and I like him, and I know she wants to look as good as possible at Melinda's wedding, so I speak up. "I'll wear that dress. It's fine. I have terrible tan lines anyway."

The tan lines are an easier excuse than the underlying reason for them. It's true the skin on my back and shoulders has cleared up along with my face, but for a while it was terrible. The last couple of summers got me in the habit of covering it up – no tank tops, rash guards for swimming – and it's hard to reverse.

"There's not much in this world as off-putting as bad tan lines," Rachel says.

I can't figure out if she's being her usual blunt self or if, knowing why I wouldn't want to wear spaghetti straps, this is her attempt to be uncharacteristically supportive. Paige was away on a residency for most of the time I was battling my skin, and Melinda was living in Vancouver with Bill while he articled. I don't think either of them are particularly aware of how bad my acne really got, or the journey it took me on.

Rachel, though, was not only in the city, but had moved back home for two months while her apartment was repaired following a major water leak. After my sobs woke her up the night Rory dumped me, she appeared in my doorway and wordlessly climbed into bed to hug me to sleep. It was Rachel who found out about Dr. Hamilton from a co-worker with a teenage daughter, and my often-caustic sister drove me to my first appointment.

I push the brochure back toward Melinda.

"All good?" she asks.

"Fine." I nod.

She sighs. "Thank goodness that's finally sorted out. Now let's talk about Saturday. We're meeting at eleven to sample small plates."

"I can't." I say it automatically because for every Saturday of my school life in recent memory, it would be true. I'd have a ringette try-out, or practice, or game.

"Why not?" Melinda asks.

Shit. Now that my brain has caught up with my mouth, I know that everybody knows I don't have ringette this Saturday. I also know I really, really don't want to go nibble shredded lobster, and spiced polenta, and gluten free cake options with my mini-bridezilla of a sister.

"I'm horseback riding."

Melinda's brow furrows. "Since when?"

"Since Em's away, and her horse needs exercising, so her coach asked me to ride him in a Learn to Ride class."

"And it's Saturday?"

I nod. "Saturday." My fingers are crossed under my seat. "Definitely Saturday."

"Well it had better not interfere with the wedding."

"Of course not. It won't. But I can't miss this weekend. Em's counting on me."

"Hmm ... well. I feel like Em should make arrangements for her own horse."

"And I feel like you can taste your own small plates," I mumble.

"Pardon me?"

"She has made arrangements. With me."

"I thought that's what you said."

***

My just-washed hair is wet – trailing down my back – and that, combined with the late evening breeze luffing through my window, raises goosebumps on my skin.

What makes a poem a poem?

The words sit above a sea of bright white on my screen.

I've started and deleted six different answers.

"Knock, knock," comes my mom's voice from the doorway.

Every night, all my life, my mom has come to this door and said, "Knock, knock." For so many years, it was, "Knock, knock my girls." We'd hear it from down the hall first, at Melinda and Rachel's door, then she'd make her way to see Paige and me.

Now it's just me left.

"Honey, you're cold." My mom trails her hand along my arm and reaches for the window. Then she stops. "Sorry. You're a big girl now. I should let you take care of yourself."

I smile. "It's OK Mom. I should close the window, or at least put on a hoodie, but it was such a hot summer, and we complained so much, I feel like I should enjoy the cool air now."

The other truth is I've always loved this time of year. The summers in our city are legendary for their record-breaking high temperatures combined with soupy humidity. Even before my acne turned truly terrible, I always thought of June through August as break-out season, as the sensitive, oily skin I could usually control in the cooler months would take on an inflamed, irritated life of its own. It's why I turned down customer-facing summer jobs and have always spent the summer landscaping. It's why I welcomed cool nights and crisp days when everyone else was lamenting the end of the summer heat.

"That's a good point." My mom crosses her arms and rubs them. "So, about this riding ...?"

"Oh. Yeah. I'm sorry." My hand automatically moves the mouse to click on the Stonegate tab open in my browser. "I couldn't face the plate-tasting."

"Was it just an excuse, then?"

I wrinkle my nose and wave toward the screen where, on one of my many procrastinating moves, I've pulled up the Learn to Ride program details. "Well, it *is* Saturday morning, but it's not cheap, and it's a half-hour drive, so yes, a temporary excuse until I come up with a better one."

My mom lays a hand on my shoulder as she stands behind me and reads. "Eight weeks ... fully certified instructor ... basics of horsemanship ... did I ever tell you I always wanted to ride?"

I turn to look at her over my shoulder. "No! I had no idea."

She nods. "That's why I always like talking to Em about her horse. Lucas. Such a nice name." Em's boyfriend Lucas grew up two houses over from us. My mom loves Lucas, and she would love any creature with his name.

"Maybe you should take the program, Mom."

"Oh, I'm past wanting to ride. But ..."

"But what?"

"But, you got that entrance scholarship, which we weren't expecting, and we're spending so much on this wedding I can't think one more charge would make such a difference – if you want to sign up for that program, Ellie, I'll pay for it."

I can be calm about this offer, because it's not real. "You work on Saturday mornings, Mom. You need the car."

"Oh, Gwyneth is always saying we should carpool. I'm sure she'll pick me up and drive me to work for eight weeks."

"But, doesn't carpooling mean you should drive sometimes? And what if she's sick?"

My mom's solved problems for all of us our whole lives. Something this simple is nothing for her. "I'll help her pay for gas and if she's sick, we'll deal with that at the time. You, or your dad can drop me off, or I can take the bus."

"Or I can miss riding." As soon as I've said it I realize I don't really want to miss it. It makes me feel the same way I'd feel if I knew I had to miss Legal Studies with Addy.

"I'm sure it won't come to that. If we can marry Melinda off in line with her very high standards, I'm sure we can get you to horseback riding eight weeks in a row."

Oh. "Oh! I ... wow ... I don't know what to say."

My mom squeezes my shoulder. "Say yes because otherwise your sister will find out you lied to her, and I wouldn't want to be you if that happens."

Chapter Five

I switch off the car engine, then just sit and stare out the windscreen.

A text pinged in when I was partway here. Now, I swipe my screen to read **Are you there yet? I'm so excited! Give Lucas a carrot for me.**

I thumb back. **I'm here. Don't want to get out of car. Feeling pretty dumb.** Then I send a photo of the rubber boots I'm wearing. They're swirled with a purple and turquoise paisley print. Come to think of it, they'd match my fancy new loose-leaf.

I follow up with **Just my luck Rachel is the only one with the same shoe size as me. Paige has normal rubber boots, but they fall off my feet.**

Do they have low heels?

Yes.

Then they're fine. All you need. Get out of the car and spoil my horse.

That's just the problem. If you don't even know how to approach a horse; if you're convinced its massive hooves are going to crush your rubber-boot-clad feet, how on earth do you even go about beginning to spoil a horse?

There are three quick taps on the passenger window and I glance up just in time to see Laney's waving arm, then her retreating back. Her "Come on!" is muffled by the closed car window.

I text Em **OK. Going.** Then drop my phone into the door pouch, and go.

***

Oh, great. Everyone else is a munchkin. *Stupid, stupid, stupid*. I'm not sure why, but it never occurred to me that I might be the only person here over ten years old.

For a second I lock eyes with a girl about my height, and I'm about to smile and go stand beside her, until she reaches out and straightens the bow in a small blond child's hair. *Oh*. She's her *mother*.

The creature tied in the aisle is so small even I know it's a pony. It's not much taller than our neighbours' Great Dane, and I feel like I could pick it up and carry it away if I really had to, but there's this glint in its eye that's very clearly saying, *Do. Not. Come. Near. Me.*

The kids don't seem to notice. They're swarming it. One girl is braiding its tail. The other one is braiding the hair that grows over its face. The boy is the only one who seems to be trying to actually clean the beast. He's using a brush to attack a patch of dried mud.

The pony stretches its face toward the braiding girl and opens its mouth and I take a half step forward and point. "It's going to bite her!"

"She," says a voice beside me.

I turn to face a girl slightly taller than the two working on the pony. I recognize her thin face and red hair from coming out here with Em. 'Fox girl,' – I can hear Em saying it, but I can't remember the real name that should go with it. "Pardon?" I ask.

"The pony's a 'she' – not an 'it' – and she won't bite. She's just sniffing."

It's true that the pony hasn't bitten the girl. *Yet.* But I'm still not sure. "Hmm ..." I say.

"You're Ellie," the girl says. "I'm Sasha, and Em and Laney told me you were coming, and I'll pull Lucas out for you."

Sasha. That's it. "Oh. Yes. We've met before ..."

She's walking away.

I duck under the tie attached to the pony and say "Excuse me," to the watching mother, and watch as Sasha leads a familiar, big horse out and secures him the same way the pony is, and I suddenly think maybe I should stick with glinty eyes and inquisitive noses, because I'd forgotten how *huge* this horse is.

I can't touch him. I can't even go near him. I'm about to say so, when Laney walks into the aisle and claps her hands together, and says, "Welcome to Session One of the Learn to Ride program. I'm so looking forward to working with all of you," and I want to also be looking forward to working with her, but right now it requires a big leap of faith to imagine how that's going to work.

***

There's a shaky moment, when we all have to try on helmets to make sure we have one that will fit us when we ride next week. Laney instructs us to tuck our hair behind our ears and snap up the harness, and I feel ridiculously vulnerable. There's a reason I wear my long hair loose whenever I can – it only gets pulled back for running. Even at home I've become used to the security of the long, thick curtain hanging beside my cheeks.

Wearing this helmet, I feel like my cheeks are out there, glowing, inviting the whole world to eyeball them. Logically, I know they're fine – smooth – but my stored memories of painful cysts, and ticking-time-bomb whiteheads are seared in my brain.

Not something you really want other people examining.

Laney and Sasha are going from person to person asking, "How does that feel?" giving the helmet some careful pokes and prods, looking for gaps. Sasha gets me to kneel on a hay bale then walks around me. When she's facing me again, she crinkles her nose, wrinkles her forehead, and says "You just have ..." She reaches a hand out. I'm holding my breath, I'm sweating. "... a bit of hair sticking straight out there." She tucks it under the harness and smiles. "Perfect! You look like a pro already."

The little kids might be holding back groans, but I'm happy when Laney claps her hands together and says, "OK, back to our horsemanship theory. As I was saying, there are three main reasons we groom our horse ..."

Because I'm a good student – or at least a diligent student – I listen carefully, paying more attention to Laney than to my surroundings, which causes me to mistakenly step back once, twice, and into range of Lucas's teeth. Which I can feel now, on the back of my neck.

Holy crap. My heart vrooms into overdrive and, for a second, I can't breathe.

OK, it's not his teeth I feel, *exactly*. It's his nose, or whatever you call that part of a horse's face. And it's so close I can feel his hot breath whiffling through my hair, and along my skin, and under my collar, and down my spine.

It makes me giggle.

And, I discover, it's impossible to be panicked while I'm giggling. I reach back and feel soft, warm, living skin – nothing hard, no teeth, nothing that could hurt me.

In fact, when Lucas loses interest in my non-carrot-scented neck, it feels cold without him snuffling it.

Sasha takes over, and bosses me through the rest of the grooming session, and before I know it we're done, and Laney's saying good-bye to everyone, and reminding us we'll be riding next Saturday. She asks Sasha, "Can you take Lucas back to the small barn with Ellie so she'll know where his stall is for next week?"

Everything Sasha does would be a trial for me. Snapping the leash – "Lead," she corrects me – onto his halter (I've learned what that's called). Guiding the strong, heavy horse through the yard where he follows her more politely than most of the neighbourhood dogs I see out for walks with their owners. Leading him safely through the narrow door of his stall, and taking his halter off.

This twelve-year-old is making me feel very inadequate.

"Em asked me to give him a carrot," I say.

Sasha nods. "Sure! Go ahead, he'll love it."

"I ... the thing is ... I have no idea how to even do that." *And I'm not sure if I want to.* Because, even though Lucas didn't use his teeth on me earlier, they're definitely involved in carrot eating.

"No problem!" Sasha says. I've decided she's not a fox. She's more of a puppy – always happy, always eager, always up for the next thing, never impatient. She takes the carrot I'm holding and snaps it in two. "First you break off a big chunk like this..."

She holds her hand out, with the half she's kept balanced on the flat of her palm, and the transaction is quick and simple. Nobody bites, nobody cries, both parties are happy with all body parts intact. "Just do the same thing I did," Sasha says.

I lift my hand, with the carrot balled inside, and Lucas's ears go forward. "Good," Sasha says, "Now you have to make it easy for him to get it. Open your hand so the carrot is sitting right there."

He's watching me with the same kind of look my sisters had for that steak my dad barbecued the other night. And I know how that went ...

"Trust him." And suddenly Sasha's hand is under mine, lifting it. Now I can't not open my hand because it will show not only that I don't trust Lucas, but that I don't trust her, either.

I open my fingers and I'm afraid the carrot's going to roll right off, but Lucas has that under control.

There's a gentle whiffling, whisking, kissing, brush of velvet over my skin and with a touch that feels like butterfly wings, the carrot is gone, and he's crunching.

"Oh!" I say.

Sasha giggles.

I turn and look at her. "How can he be so gentle?"

"Believe it or not, if you add powdered supplements to their grain, horses can actually pick them out and eat around them. So taking a carrot off your hand ... no big deal."

"Wow," I say.

Wow. I know I learned a lot today – most of which I'll probably forget by next week – but this seems big. This seems huge.

This horse doesn't want to hurt me and he doesn't care how I do things – he's happy as long as he gets the carrot in the end.

I might not know anything else about looking after this horse ... I might have no clue how to get from the ground to his back ... but I can bring carrots every week.

No problem there.

I'm going to add them to the shopping list as soon as I get home.

Chapter Six

I avoided the small plates tasting session, but I can't avoid the after-discussion when we all meet for Sunday dinner at Melinda's.

"So we're going to do this scientifically," Melinda says. She's printed off a chart with names typed across the top – **Free Range Bison Medallions with Pancetta and Morels, Chorizo Filled Dates Wrapped in Prosciutto, Sea Bass Ceviche** and more – and we're each given a bingo dabber. "You each get three small plates votes and two dessert votes. Just use your dabber to make a mark under the dishes you liked best."

My sisters press forward and Melinda yells, "Stop!" She holds her hand out to me. "Except Ellie, since she didn't come to the tasting. Surrender the dabber."

I smack it into her hand and mutter. "Fine with me. I'd have to Google half those ingredients anyway."

The scientific food selection proceeds with Sea Bass Ceviche coming out a clear favourite and Melinda axing it from the list. "Hey!" Rachel protests. "We all loved that!"

"Hmm ..." Melinda says. "Well, I think it's messy and, anyway, half the time caterers substitute in cheaper fish without you knowing it, so I'm taking it off."

"But you said it was a scientific decision."

Melinda's eyebrows lift. "Obviously the bride gets a veto."

Our dinner is very good. Chili cooked by Melinda's fiancé, Bill, who never uses ingredients that require Googling.

I eat, and let my head fill with Lucas – I can see now that Em is right that he has very cute ears – and quiz myself on details like, *What are the three reasons for grooming?* and *What is the right order to use the grooming brushes?*

It passes the time while my sisters debate the merits of pancetta over prosciutto, but it means I'm caught completely off guard when the next topic arises, and don't realize I'm right in the middle of the discussion until I notice the buzz around the table has died away and everybody's looking at me.

I swallow a mouthful of chili and say, "Sorry – what?"

"The seating chart." From her tone, I can tell Melinda's already said this at least twice.

"Oh. Yeah. OK. Just put me wherever. I'm easy." I smile. There – I'm not causing a problem – they can let me go back to trying to remember the name of that funny "v" thing in Lucas's foot.

"Ellie ..." Clearly I'm not off the hook. "Are you bringing anybody?"

For some reason I look at my mom, even though it's not like she has the answer. She is, however, really good at sticking up for me when my sisters overwhelm me, and I'm afraid no matter what answer I give they're going to do just that.

"Yes," will lead to a barrage of questions about *Who?* Is it somebody important? Is it somebody I'm dating? Plus, it would then put me under pressure to actually produce said person.

I suspect "no" would also be wrong. Something about not taking Melinda's wedding seriously, or an in-depth scrutiny of my social life.

Usually their conversation moves on pretty quickly, but everyone's still quiet – still looking at me – so I say, "Um ... hmm ... probably not?"

"Um!" Rachel states hers with confidence and oomph. "Yes, she is."

All eyes swing to Rachel, but she's looking right at me. "Of course you are. I'm sorry, Ellie, you're in your first year of university, you're young, you're pretty, you're single. You should have fun. You won't have fun if you come without a guest; you'll spend the night dancing with our eight-year-old cousins and Bill's perverted old Uncle Bob – sorry, Bill – both of whom will step on your toes, and

Melinda will make you run around and check all the flowers to remove any that are wilting, and you'll end up being the designated driver for lushy old Aunt Matilda ..." Rachel makes an I-rest-my-case gavel motion, and says. "It'll be the suckiest of all sucky weddings."

Don't look at Melinda. Not that I have to – I can guarantee the word "sucky" uttered in the same sentence as "wedding" has triggered her eyes to turn to laser beams that will kill anyone who makes the mistake of making eye contact.

Instead I focus on Rachel. "You don't sound sorry."

Next to me, Paige chokes and a chunk of cornbread falls to her plate. "Oh, my goodness. Excuse me," she says.

"Listen." The steel in Melinda's voice makes it clear that we are done with diversions. That *she* is done with diversions, which means the rest of us had better be, too. "If you're not bringing anyone, there's time for me to send out one extra invite ..."

Cue my protector Mom. "Melinda ..."

"What?"

"You know what."

My sister shakes her head, but Melinda knows my normally mild mother does have a breaking point which my sister is skating perilously close to. Her next words are a mutter. "Whatever. We'll talk about it later."

***

Later finds me home, in my room, trying to prop my eyes open long enough to finish the French play I'm supposed to have read for tomorrow's class.

It is *not* riveting.

But I'm trying really hard to avoid the pointless time-wasting of click-click-clicking around social media sites. I gave myself fifteen minutes to spend on them tonight, and as proof of just how boring this play is, I used my time up during Act II.

Email. Email isn't social media. I make myself a deal – finish two more scenes, which will leave me with just a few pages left to read tomorrow, which I can easily do before class.

Two more scenes and I can check my email, then go to bed. It's a plan.

I finally, *finally* read the last sentence, force myself to think back over the scene I just finished to make sure I actually understand it, then I close my book. Thank goodness.

Interspersed between all the usual junk emails are the few that make me smile. One from Em with a couple of short video clips attached. **I snuck into Lucas's basketball practice at college today. Doesn't he look good in his practice pinney?**

I watch the videos. Type back. **Nice form! And, unlike you, I'm talking about his shooting form. Say hi to him for me.**

One from Addy. **Here's the thing – I can't read my own handwriting on the stuff we covered about the constitution. Honestly, look at the attachment. Can you help?**

I open what looks like a picture of hieroglyphics. *Whoa.* **Remind me never to be sick and ask you for notes. See attached. If you need a better look I can show you in class.** I snap pictures of a couple of my pages of notes and attach them.

There's one I save for last. It has a familiar subject line. **Once my patient ... always my patient.** It's from Dr. Hamilton – another way she's different from other doctors. She sends newsletters celebrating her patients and their successes.

For a long time I was too afraid to ask my family doctor about my skin – I figured it was right there for her to see, and she'd tell me if it was a problem. Then, when I experienced what I thought was the worst break-out of my life except it showed no signs of going away, I finally made an appointment to ask about it. She told me she didn't like to go overboard on what she considered to be a cosmetic problem, and prescribed a seemingly endless string of topical treatments, some of which actually made my acne worse.

When Rachel told me we were calling Dr. Hamilton I wasn't sure what to think. What could another doctor do that my first doctor hadn't? And wasn't I just overreacting – being vain – when other people had much bigger problems?

But Dr. Hamilton was different from day one. Told me about her own teenage struggle with acne. About how she grew up in a small northern community and had to drive four hours for each skin appointment. Talked about how exhausting it was to keep smiling and going to school, and to her job as a lifeguard, all while hating the way she looked, and feeling the actual physical pain of her acne, and how she never wanted anyone else to go through what she did.

Said she would help me.

It's no exaggeration to say she changed my life, which is why when her newsletters come out I read every word. They're direct and positive, just like her.

Today's newsletter links to some new research into the comorbidity of acne and depression. It has a picture of the new therapy dog Dr. Hamilton has adopted to replace the former therapy dog who just retired to live with one of her former patients. It has my favourite part – the patient highlight story. This month it's about a former patient who just fulfilled her goal of being hired on as a firefighter. The story isn't about her skin – it's about the challenges she had to overcome to get where she is. It's about her hopes for the future. There's a picture of her – beaming and clear-skinned – in her firefighting uniform.

As usual there's Dr. Hamilton's tagline at the bottom of the newsletter, **Once my patient, always my patient** then in small, hyperlinked letters, **Unless you want to unsubscribe, in which case just click here!** I can't imagine ever clicking that link.

I close my laptop and go to the bathroom to brush my teeth and wash my face. I stare into the mirror – the same one I used to lean into to examine the latest eruption on my face, to decide whether I could actually leave the house – and it shows me clear-skinned, lightly freckled, with a bloom of colour in my cheeks. Normal. It shows me normalcy.

I can see it; I just can't quite feel it.

Yet. I tell myself. I don't feel it *yet*. As always when I get one of Dr. Hamilton's letters I resolve to try harder, to put myself out there, to appreciate the gift she's giving me and do something with it.

Chapter Seven

Although every day the trees sport more and more red, and yellow, and orange leaves, and the nights are quite crisp, the days are sunny and mild with a hazy kind of autumn mist hanging in the air. I keep cycling to school – putting off the day when I'll have to rely on the bus, standing in the crowded aisles, snugging my backpack at my feet to avoid hitting other passengers with it.

I'm getting used to my schedule. Starting to know what I need to bring to campus with me. Beginning to recognize other people who have schedules that intersect with mine at certain regular touchpoints.

There's the older woman with sparkling silver hair (a professor?) who locks her upright commuter bike one rack over from mine at least two mornings a week. The guy I recognize from my high school who wears a different bright-coloured turban every day – I always pass him while he's standing in a line-up for his coffee. And there's another guy I've noticed half-a-dozen times. He has to be on the basketball team. It's not just his height – it's the general impression of total and complete athleticism he gives off. Oh, and the logo on his long, loose shorts which identifies them as coming from the same competitive club both Lucas and Rory played for.

Then there's my sister.

The wonder whiz of the university fundraising community.

Although Rachel will often mutter that she didn't get her MBA to beg rich people for money, they love her here. Her rise in the development department is meteoric, and the university has announced they've exceeded their funding targets for a new library since they hired her.

Seeing her clacking along the commons in her power heels with her shiny auburn hair twisted into a let's-get-down-to-business bun, I hardly recognize her.

Rachel's always a little bit scary, but here, at her place of work – the place where she's a runaway success – she's borderline terrifying.

"Ellie!" She yells and I freeze. So do the six or so students caught between the two of us. The girls sidestep casually out of the way as my sister advances toward me. One of the guys looks at her, then away, then does what I can only describe as scurrying. The second guy stares openly – Rachel does rock a pencil skirt – she turns to him and says, "Take a picture; it'll last longer," before threading her arm through mine and saying, "Come on, sis, falafel I think!"

Which is how, two weeks in a row, I've ended up eating lunch with Rachel. She's generous ... to a point. She'll buy my lunch, but only if I eat what she wants.

Week one is falafel, week two is fish tacos. "How about the veggie bowl place?" I ask.

Rachel shakes her head as she runs her finger through a glop of crema on her plate. "No can do."

"Why not?"

She waggles her eyebrows. "I had a thing with the guy who runs it."

"Oh." I should be used to this kind of thing with Rachel, but her easy casualness always catches me off guard. "It didn't go well?"

She licks her finger. "It was fine – better than average, if I'm honest. But I don't want him to get any ideas. I mean I can't have a long-term relationship with a guy who constantly smells like fried onions. How about you?"

What I want to ask is, *How do you do it?* and a little bit, *How would I even take the first step?* What I say is, "I like fried onions."

"Oh for God's sake, Ellie. Not onions. A guy. Some guy. Any guy. Or a girl, if you prefer. A *partner*, I guess, if we're being politically correct."

I'm about to say, *Don't trouble yourself to be politically correct*, when a girl's voice chimes up. "Ellie?" I turn, and Addy says, "Oh! It is you. I'm so glad. The only empty table

is next to these guys playing with their condiments –
which, don't get me wrong, I used to think was a totally
fun thing to do … when I was seven – and then I saw you
over here at this primo table …"

We do have a good table. It's in the window, overlook-
ing a green stretch leading down to the river. Rachel gave
the two women sitting here a look, and they cleared away
pronto saying "We were just going!"

"Thanks," Rachel had said and sat down before they
were even done removing their plates.

The sleek, gorgeous, super-pro version of my sister
looks up and down at Addy sporting yet another pair of
overalls – these ones with purple piping on the straps and
the front pocket – her hair in French braids, and a pair of
funky tortoiseshell glasses, and pulls out the chair next to
her. "Have a seat."

I'm equal parts happy and worried that Rachel and
Addy hit it off. On the surface they might look different,
but it only takes two minutes to notice how Addy's effer-
vescent sparkle packs just as much punch as Rachel's
unrelenting energy.

When Addy mentions the extra credit she's added to
her timetable, Rachel nods. "I did that too. It let me start
grad school a semester early."

Rachel's happy to give Addy advice on extra-curricu-
lars. "These are the ones that will look really good on your

transcript," and even mentions. "The fundraising office hires students a few times a year. If you give me your email I can let you know when we're hiring if you think you might want a part-time job."

A part-time job? Do days have twenty-five hours in Addy's world? I have no idea how she already manages everything she's doing, but she beams. "Great, thanks," as she thumbs her contact information into my sister's phone.

Their mutual liking is good for obvious reasons.

The worry kicks in as soon as Rachel says, "Just before you got here Ellie and I were discussing her love-life. You two aren't, you know, interested in each other, are you?"

I smack my forehead with my hand. "Oh. My. God. Rachel, you cannot go around asking things like that!"

My sister opens her eyes as round and wide as a baby owl and says, "Why not? I'm just making sure everybody's on the same page."

Addy laughs. "I wish I could fall for someone like your sister. Instead I have a pathetically long-lasting unrequited crush on a guy who a) has asked my younger sister out half-a-dozen times, b) called me 'Abby' all through high school on the rare occasions he actually addressed me, and c) wrote in the yearbook that he wants to be a plastic surgeon because he'll be able to get rich by touching women's breasts."

I nudge Rachel. "This is where you tell her she could do way, way better than that."

Rachel's nodding, though. "He's got 'it' doesn't he?"

Addy nods. "In spades.

Rachel shrugs. "Been there, done that."

Addy laughs. "But I bet you at least got to buy the t-shirt."

"Usually the t-shirt's not all it's cracked up to be," Rachel says. Then adds, "And, of course you could do better. But at least you have your heart set on someone, unlike my sister."

Addy's eyebrows fly up. "There's nobody?"

First instinct: *deflect*. Change the subject. Don't discuss something that could be embarrassing.

Until I remember. Rachel's the one who drives me to my dermatologist. Addy and I have already discussed our unfortunate condition-in-common. If I can't talk to them ...

I shrug. "OK, let me tell you about getting dumped. When I started dating my best friend's brother ..."

Addy throws up her hand. "Let me stop you right there. That is a very bad idea." She turns to Rachel. "Isn't it?"

Rachel does a half nod, half head shake. "I mean, yeah, but I once dated my dad's boss, so ..."

My spine shoots ramrod straight, "You, what?!?"

"Never mind," Rachel says. "It's a story for another day. Besides, it was less 'dating' more …"

I stick my fingers in my ears. "No, no, no … I do not want to know!" When my sister's lips stop moving, I resume my Rory tale. "Anyway, when we started dating my skin was OK. I mean, not great, but fine. Then …" I shrug. "… I have no idea what happened, but it got *bad*. Really quickly. Which, I accept, isn't what he expected, but it also wasn't what I expected."

I take a sip of my drink. "I'm going to give him an A for effort on the break-up. He tried hard. I think he Googled 'how to break up.' He used a combination of the 'it's not you, it's me' and the shit-sandwich techniques. Started with how much he liked me … *at first* …" I throw in the biggest eye roll I can and Addy sits back in her chair, takes a handful of organic popcorn and says, "This should be good …"

I nod. "If by good, you mean terrible." I give an exaggerated exhale before resuming. "Then he said it was his problem for not being attracted to me anymore, and he didn't know why, but he just didn't see me the same way as he used to, and he wanted to be honest with me to avoid any bitterness."

"Ouch," Addy says. "And was he staring at your biggest whitehead the whole time?"

Addy astounds me with her openness. Up until now even hearing the word "zit" out loud was enough to give me hives. It's strange, but nice, to be able to actually talk about something I've held in for so long. *Go along with it.* "I had two doozies that day. I don't think he knew where to look."

Addy flicks her eyes from my chest to Rachel's. "Sorry, ladies, I just can't decide which of your breasts to stare at." She lifts her fingers and makes air quotes. "Boy problems."

She drops her hands. "What about now, though? Look how gorgeous you are. You can show him."

"Very good question." Rachel holds her fist out for a bump, and Addy obliges.

"This was a big first step for me," I protest. "Talking about it."

"Talking about it is not going to get you laid," Addy says.

Rachel starts gathering up her food wrap. "Don't worry. I've already told her she's bringing someone to our sister's wedding, so she has a deadline to work to." She shakes a mint into her palm and offers them around. "And, no offense Addy; as much as I like you, I don't want to see you on Ellie's arm at the wedding."

Addy takes a mint. "No worries. I will *not* be your sister's plus one."

Chapter Eight

Half-an-hour early. That's what Laney said. Only somehow I added half-an-hour to my original half-an-hour. Our lesson starts at 11:00, so I put it in my mind that I had to be there at 10:30, and then I added half-an-hour to that.

So I'm sitting in an otherwise-empty parking lot not having any idea what to do. If this was an ice rink, I'd just make myself at home. Watch whatever team was on the ice. Or stretch. Or both at the same time.

I don't know how things work at stables, though. Is it OK to get out and wander around? Will somebody tell me off?

It's not warm today, either. There were frost warnings overnight. The air in the car is cooling by the second.

I'm not a coffee drinker, but maybe I should head out to the nearest small town and look for a coffee shop. Get a tea, or a hot chocolate, or something.

Kill some time.

That's probably the thing to do.

If only I'd brought my Legal Studies textbook. If only …

Tap-tap-tap! The sharp knuckles-on-window tapping jumps my heart into double-time rhythm.

I fumble, can't find the window button. When I do, realize it won't work because I've turned the engine off.

Oh, what the ... I push the door open. "Hey Sasha."

"Hey! Oh, it's so great you're here early. You wanna help me muck out the small barn and we can bring Lucas over to the big barn together?"

Do I? "What's 'muck out?'"

"Oh! *Clean.* The stalls. And then sweep the aisle, of course, otherwise the barn looks like a huge mess."

She's already walking and I'm walking with her. She stops dead and I run into her. "Do you need anything? From the car? Because we probably won't come back."

"Um ..."

"Like is that a warm enough jacket? You'll warm up when you're riding, but it'll be cold at first – and you're wearing leggings, so those are fine, and low-heeled boots, so you're good! OK, let's go!"

I'm dizzy even though it's Sasha who should be out of breath. Just because she hasn't inhaled or exhaled doesn't mean I can't, but my body didn't get that memo.

It's been a long, long time since I've done something I know nothing about. I mean, at first I didn't know what to expect when I went out for the school cross-country and track teams, but I knew I was a decent runner. And, yeah, university is a big step, but it's still school. I already know how to take notes, write essays, study for tests.

This, though ... as I stand in the doorway looking into the little barn, somebody could point a gun at my head and say, "Muck out this barn," and the best I'd be able to do would be ... nothing at all.

Thank goodness for Sasha.

"OK, here. This is the good pitchfork and I'll give it to you because I'm used to the wonky one, so it works fine for me."

It's the first time I've ever held a pitchfork in my life. I didn't know it was possible to have a "good" vs. "wonky" version.

"Only two of the stalls in here are being used right now, and my pony, Oreo ..." Sasha points to the stall on the right, "... is out with the herd, so we'll just put Lucas on the cross-ties and we'll be good to go."

"Hey-buddy-hey-boy-hey-Lukey-Lukey-Lukey-hi-pretty-boy-hi-silly ..." She leads the horse out of his stall – he hasn't gotten any smaller since the last time I saw him – and positions him in a particular spot, and says, "Can you just do up the cross-tie on that side?" and I remember the cross-tie is the rope that hangs from high up on the wall, and I find it, and click it on the ring on Lucas's halter (*I remembered it was called a halter!*) and I feel a ridiculous flare of pride.

Sasha manoeuvres a wheelbarrow much bigger than her into a spot equidistant from the two stall doors, and says, "Cool! Let's go." She picks up her sub-standard pitchfork and walks into Oreo's stall and says, "It's really simple – you just find all the poop and chuck it in the barrow," a barrage of plump brown balls fly through the air to make a satisfying sound against the thick plastic bucket of the wheelbarrow, and Lucas watches, ears pricked forward, the way I've seen Rory and Lucas watch NCAA basketball players make free throws.

"Also," Sasha continues, "You take out all the shavings that are wet – you can tell because they're dark and dirty-looking – then you just heap the clean shavings in banks around the edges of the stall until the whole middle is bare and clean, then call me."

I realize this isn't rocket-science – and, after all, I'm an intelligent person attending university on a scholarship – but it's new, and different, and I'm afraid I won't be any good at it. Still, the twelve-year-old is doing it, so ...

I pick up my premium pitchfork, step into the stall, and select a nice, clear mound of manure. My toss gets about half of it into the wheelbarrow.

I keep going, imagining a grid super-imposed on the stall floor that I have to work my way through. It's unexpectedly, deeply satisfying. I'm determined not to leave a single dirty shaving in Lucas's stall, while, at the same time setting myself the personal goal of throwing out few-to-no clean ones.

I fall into a rhythm – *scan, pick, shake, toss* and *bank, fluff, pile.*

Soon the centre of the stall is bare, and each wall has a hill of shavings piled against it.

"Nice!"

I turn to face Sasha, surveying my stall-cleaning efforts. I'm absurdly proud. "Is it good?" I know it is, I just want her to say it.

"It's excellent! Now, next steps ..."

She shows me how to re-fluff the bedding around the stall – "We hardly have to put in any new shavings because you were so careful when you mucked out," – my chest puffs out when she says that, and when we're done the stall looks and smells dry, and clean, and comfortable.

"I think I'd sleep in here," I say.

"A good horsewoman always puts her horse first."

"I hardly know anything about horses," I say.

Sasha taps her head. "Being a horse person is a state of mind." She sweeps her arm around the finished stall. "I'd say you've got it."

***

There are four of us lined up in the ring and I have a straight view across to Laney because all the others are holding small ponies. Big, lumbering Lucas and I stand at the end.

"I'm going to come around and help you all with your stirrups and girths, and then we'll get everybody up and riding!" Laney says.

I cast a sideways glance at Lucas. "Up" is right.

It looks like I'll be last, and that's OK with me. I'm used to Lucas now – from the ground – he's a large, quiet, restful presence. I've come to believe he doesn't want to hurt me and I'm reluctant to disturb that balance by climbing up on his back.

I run my fingers along the crest of his neck. "We can wait, right buddy?"

"I can help you!"

Sasha.

"Of course you can."

"Yeah – of course I can! Laney wants to work with the little kids, and that's fine with me, because they're a pain anyway ... but I can get you going." She steps up beside me. "Let me show you how to figure out how long your stirrup should be ..."

After manipulating a lot of buckles on long straps of leather, Sasha assures me the saddle is secure, and won't twist under Lucas's belly (which is an eventuality that had never even occurred to me before she mentioned it) and she walks in front of me toward a big step-like thing she

THROW YOUR HEART OVER

calls the mounting block, saying over her shoulder, "Next week, you can do all that stuff yourself, but it's good to get you going today."

Oh yeah. For sure. Next week I'll most definitely know exactly how to put the right buckle on the right strap and tighten it to the right tension. Not a problem.

"Just bring him up beside here … no Lucas, come on, you know better." There's grunting and clucking from the far side of the big horse and he takes some small steps, and Sasha pops up from behind him and says, "Perfect! Now you just climb up!"

"Climb up?"

"Yeah, climb up to the top of the block there, and it should be really easy for you to just put your leg over and you're good to go!"

The twelve-year-old says to do it, so I guess I should do it.

"Come on," Sasha says. "Put your left foot in the stirrup, like this, and just swing over his back … there!"

And I'm sitting on Lucas's back.

Sasha is puttering around at the level of my feet, doing more of her strap fiddling, and yanking, and adjusting, and there's no doubt she's going to have to repeat all of it next week because no part of me is paying any attention.

I'm just looking down at the strong hump in front of the saddle that Laney and Sasha both told me was called the withers. It's one of those funny plural words for a single thing. From there I can see how Lucas's body flows to his strong shoulders, and looking up again it's amazing to have his long strong neck stretched in front of me.

"OK, Ellie?" Sasha's shading her eyes as she looks up at me and I have no idea what she was saying, but Lucas turns his head, and gives my toe a gentle bump, followed by a soft snuffling exhale and to me, it's like he's saying, "I'm here," and "I'm not going anywhere," and "I'll take care of you," and, since those are exactly the things I want to hear, I smile at Sasha and say, "Yeah. Of course. OK."

***

I suppose we don't do much riding, but it's enough for me.

The three other riders in the lesson are all members of the tween-and-under crowd and are all accompanied by their parents – correction: *mothers* – let's face it, horseback riding seems to be more of a motherly occupation.

While I was jealous before that all these small kids got to ride small ponies, I'm starting to see the benefits of riding Lucas instead.

He's steady, calm … *sane.*

He walks forward politely along the track in the ring – Sasha calls it the rail; it's one of the many things she chit-chats about as she walks alongside Lucas. But not touching him.

Whatever level of riding this is that I'm doing, I'm doing it myself. I'm proud of that.

Especially as I watch the other three.

True, one is doing fine. That particular pony marches along the rail with his head at the waist height of a mother even I find quite scary. She's tall, solidly built, has a firm grasp on the pony's lead and, as I watch, he sways sideways and she bumps him back into line with her hip. After that his tail swishes occasionally – "Is he angry?" I ask Sasha, "Or is he swishing at a fly?"

Sasha laughs. "Oh, he's mad – see how his ears pin back when he flicks his tail? He's really lazy and that lady is making him walk." The lady in question swings her gaze our way for a quick second, and both Sasha and I gulp.

"She is scary," I whisper. Her little girl doesn't seem to notice, though. She might not be learning much about steering her own pony but she's singing and knocking her hands on her helmet, and seems happy enough.

Unlike the other two child riders. One's still firmly marooned in the middle of the ring where Laney left him after adjusting all his straps and moving onto the second pony-rider combo. That pair is now randomly weaving around the ring, with the girl riding him yelling, "Whoa! No ... go!" and her mother trailing behind them like a ribbon tied to the end of a string of an escaping helium balloon.

They trot past us and Lucas inclines his ear slightly in their direction while not moving off his course even an inch. Sasha calls to the mother or the girl – I'm not sure which one – "You have to be firm with him – he needs to know you're in charge!" and Laney traipses toward the recalcitrant pony who, upon seeing her approaching decides it's time to move forward and walk out of the centre of the ring.

"What do you think?" I realize Sasha's attention has refocused away from the disobedient pony back to me.

"Um, I think he's a really good boy."

She smiles and reaches out to pat Lucas's neck. Briefly. I'm still riding him alone. "He's great. And you look good on him. Your hips are following very well."

They are? I hadn't even thought about my hips. Now, for a few long, smooth strides, I do. Maybe I see what Sasha means – every time Lucas uses one of his legs, a movement travels up and into my body. Because he's been so well-behaved, I've stayed relaxed and, I guess, that means my hips are following him.

Wow. I'm good. I'm riding by myself and my hips are doing exactly what they should be.

"Your heels on the other hand ..." Sasha says.

"What? What about my heels?"

"They're up again. Push them down. Number one basic of riding."

Oh. I push my heels down.

"Twice as far as that," Sasha says.

I stick my tongue out at her and she shrugs. "You want me to tell you what's wrong with how you're holding your reins now?"

"OK, no, no ..." I push my heels down farther. There. Hopefully that'll do.

***

Back in the car the light on my phone's blinking to indicate a text from Em: **How'd it go? Dying to hear.**

I chucked out Lucas's stall.

Mucked, maybe?

Yeah, that's it. Sasha showed me how.

Impressive, but the riding – you rode today, right?

Apparently my hips are ace and my heels suck.

Anyone can learn to push their heels down, but some people never get the hip thing. You're a natural!

I'll do better with the heels next week.

Next week. Is it weird that I haven't even left the parking lot yet and I'm already looking forward to next week?

Chapter Nine

I'm trying – I really am – to write my Beowulf essay. I see the magic of the poem. It's just that right now I can't get inspired to say anything about it.

I finally had to move to the kitchen because I was afraid if I stayed in my room I wouldn't be capable of fighting the intense urge to curl up in a ball on my bed and let sleep take me away.

I'm no more motivated down here.

Maybe I've picked the wrong topic.

Maybe I started with the wrong argument.

Maybe …

"I am *so* bored!"

My sister, Rachel, thumps a bag on the counter. "Voila, the obligatory Primitive Elements, artisanal black-olive-and-caper boule. Fourteen dollars' worth. Melinda had better be happy."

I glance up. "Yeah, fourteen dollars is hella-steep for a … well, it's not even quite a loaf, is it?"

"Oh, God, Ellie. It's not the money. It's the quest required to get it."

She hooks a glass out of the cupboard and runs it full of water.

"First, I had to park, like, three kilometres from the Farmer's Market, because all the streets around it are jammed with massive black SUVs that all look the same – how on earth they ever find their cars again, I have no idea."

I smother a giggle at the mental image of my sister's acid green bubble of a car shining out from a line of near-identical sport utility vehicles.

"Then, I have to walk on the edge of the road half the time, because as if I can get by all these super-skinny women wearing four-hundred-dollar yoga pants, pushing strollers – I mean, they're not really strollers, are they, though? They're mini versions of the SUVs – they have suspension and off-road tires with leather seats and media players."

"They have media players?"

"Well. Practically."

"You're super-skinny Rach."

"I know. But I'm still naturally skinny. And ..." she holds up a hank of hair, "... naturally blonde. Nature doesn't want you to be a size two and to have Barbie blonde hair after you've given birth. I mean, really, who has time to fight gravity, bulge, and dark roots once they have kids running around?"

"You know that's in your future, Rach."

She laughs. "I know. I can pretend I like the sound of going au naturel, but when push comes to shove, I'll probably drop all the cash I can on a personal trainer and a smokin' set of highlights, too." She gulps a mouthful of tap water and I figure when she's a high-maintenance SUV-driving wife-and-mother she won't touch the stuff unless it's gone through five filters first. "Anyway, I still haven't even told you about my adventures in the bread line."

"Tell me, then."

"OK, well I finally got there, and it was snaking past all the other stands – you know the ones selling natural deodorant ..." She holds her nose with one hand and makes a waving motion with the other one to show me what she thinks of the efficacy of natural deodorant, "... and aprons made from reclaimed underwear ..."

I knit my brow and she sighs. "Well, something like that. Maybe it was ponchos made from old socks. The point is, the line was lo-o-ong and it was completely blocking access to the kale-and-quinoa lady, and everyone around me was muttering, 'They're going to run out of the black-olive-and-caper bread.' This couple in front of me was having a full-on domestic – 'I told you we should have come earlier,' and 'If you didn't take forty-five minutes in the bathroom,' and 'If you weren't out drinking until 2:00 a.m.' And, the thing is, they *were* running out of the olive bread – I could see the basket was almost empty."

She pauses for breath then continues. "Remember how Melinda freaked out the time Paige bought potato-and-dill by mistake? Luckily, I noticed one of the students who works in the fundraising office lined up ahead of me and I offered to give her a twenty and let her keep the change if she got me an olive boule."

"You don't get much change from a twenty at Primitive Elements."

Rachel shrugs. "Yeah, well, university students. It's enough for a pint, so she took it, and the domestic couple started freaking out – all 'You can't do that,' and 'That's not fair,' and the student – Lucy – said 'You want to outbid her? I'll buy you a boule for twenty-five bucks,' and they were like, 'No!' and she said, 'I thought so.'" Rachel swipes the back of her hand across her mouth. "So I got the olive bread, and Melinda won't kill me."

"I'm surprised you didn't just get there earlier and miss the whole circus and save yourself twenty bucks."

My sister grins. "Well, let's just say I was otherwise occupied this morning, and it was worth way more than twenty dollars, and it made my encounters with hipster-vegan-organic zombies almost bearable."

"The lawyer?" I ask. "The one you met in the court-house when you went to fight your ticket?"

She nods. "None other."

"He's old, though, I thought."

"He's a triathlete. Full Ironman distance – not the wussy half. The man has muscles. And endurance. And a high pain threshold ..."

"OK! OK! Enough. Are you bringing him to Melinda's wedding?"

"Seriously Ellie? The wedding is *weeks* away. As if I know who I want to bring. Although ..." She fixes me with an intense look. "I will definitely be bringing *someone*."

I drop my highlighter – which I have so far used to highlight exactly nothing – to the table. "You say it like it's just that easy."

"Ellie ..." She yanks me to my feet, pulls me into the front hall, positions me in front of the mirror. Once there, she pushes my hair forward so it spills over my shoulders, lifts it and lets it tousle into a messy-soft frame around my face. "Look. See. It *is* just that easy."

I accept that in this moment, within the tight borders of the front hall mirror, I look pretty good.

I also know how quickly that perception fades when I get out into the real world.

"You're telling me if I look pretty I can nab a partner? That's not very enlightened of you."

Rachel sighs. "It's not the worst thing in the world to go on a date with someone because you like the look of them – if it's fun, do it again. If not, at least you tried. Also …"

"Also, what?"

"Also, I knew Rory hurt your feelings, but I didn't know the details until you told Addy and me."

"And?"

"And, have you ever considered he was telling the truth?"

I break the eye contact we've established in the mirror, then resume it again. "What do you mean?"

She shrugs. "He wouldn't be the first guy to be confused about sex and relationships and what he wants. When he said it was him that stopped being attracted to you, maybe that's exactly true."

I bite my lip and Rachel says, "Oh, see how pretty you are when you do that?" She gives my hair an extra lift-fluff.

She leans in, and in the mirror her lips are so close my ear I can't see any space between us. "There's not much wrong with you, Ellie – don't go thinking there is. You've got so much to offer. You've got looks and brains."

My mind's ticking furiously with Rachel's re-interpretation of my failed relationship. Could she be right? It's too much to process right now. I sigh. "Honestly, my brains feel like mush. I can*not* get a handle on that Beowulf essay."

She waves her hand. "I can't believe they still have you doing that Beowulf essay. You and I are going out to do something fun together and it won't be about school or about men."

"No men sounds good."

"Well, actually, maybe this most recent man. He did this thing ..."

"Rach! No!"

"Shit. Sorry. Come on. I'll drive. Where do you want to go?"

***

We end up at a tack store. I've been here once before – I came with Em to pick up one of Lucas's blankets she'd brought in for professional cleaning after her previous attempt to wash horse blankets at the laundromat didn't end well.

That other time we stayed in the "horse" section of the shop. It was full of baffling items, made either of leather or of very bright nylon, with lots of buckles. I assumed horse people knew what they were for, and how to fit them on their horses, but it just put me deeper in awe of horse owners. How did you ever learn all this stuff?

This time Rachel steers me straight to the other side of the shop – an area I barely noticed the first time – the lighting is dimmer, and it's carpeted. There are strategically placed full-length mirrors. And there are racks, and racks, and racks of clothes. Hanging on rails lining the walls are – again – items I'm not that familiar with. I mean I can see they're jackets, and blouses, and riding pants, but I don't really relate to ever having a reason to wear any of them.

Despite having never touched a horse in her entire life, Rachel has the measure of this place in no time flat. "Here," she tells me. "You want to look at these racks on the inside. This is where they're showing the trendy, lifestyle stuff. Equestrian-themed, but not hardcore. Like this adorable sweater!"

The sweater she holds up would look great on my aforementioned still naturally skinny, still naturally blonde sister. "You should try it on," I say.

"Hmm ... maybe I will – it actually doesn't cost that much more than the bread – but we're here to fit you out. Come on – what do you need?"

"I ..." I look around. Shrug. "I'm not sure. My leggings and rubber boots have been OK so far."

"Well, they're actually *my* rubber boots, and I'm going to want them back at some point, so we'll have to replace those. But right now, why don't you try a pair of these?" She's holding up what initially just look like black leggings, but on closer inspection they have leather knee patches, and a reinforced cuff at the ankles and there's an actual waistband with belt loops and a snap.

I reach for them. "They actually feel quite stretchy."

Rachel nods. "These are perfect because, look, they're on super-sale and even if you quit riding, you can still wear them with a sweater and they'll look just like regular-but-even-cooler leggings."

I'm not quitting riding. The thought zips into my head so fast and furious it surprises me. I've only been on a horse once – and only at the walk – but I want to keep going. My sister's right, though. Once I shimmy into the pants which I vaguely remember Em calling "breeches" and tug and twist them into place, they do look like regular-but-even-cooler leggings, and I could wear them to school, but I can also see how they're much more durable than the thin jersey bottoms I've been wearing to the barn.

I step out of the changing room to face my sister, nodding at me and, standing next to her, a salesperson, also nodding.

I'm going to end up spending money today.

***

It's better than I expected. Turns out they sell second-hand riding gear on consignment and, turns out, there's a pair of boots my size, which means I'm able to get good quality used leather boots for the same price as the "leather-look" new ones.

Even with the good price, I hesitate, but my sister pushes in. "Listen, they look amazing on you, it's a miracle they have them in your size, you can wear them for a whole bunch of stuff – not just riding – and they're going to be my birthday present to you."

"But … my birthday isn't for ages."

"They're an early birthday present."

This is Rachel to a "t." Pushy, brash, blunt, sometimes harsh, and generous, supportive, and thoughtful. For a fleeting second an ache blooms in my chest and I blink hard. "Well, if you're sure, then, thank you."

She taps me on the head. "Just don't try to weasel another gift out of me when the time comes. This is your lot."

"Yes ma'am."

"And there is one condition."

Of course there is … "You want your rubber boots back?" There's a lift of hope at the end of my question. If only it could be that simple.

"That's not a condition, Ellie, that goes without saying. No, the condition is, since we have the same size feet, and I really quite adore these boots, if you don't bring somebody to Melinda's wedding, the boots are mine."

"What? That's not fair."

She puts her hands on her hips and says. "How is that not fair? I'm not threatening to withhold food or shelter from you; just a pair of boots you can totally live without. The deal is clear – take them on my terms, or don't take them at all."

The truth is, I've already pictured myself mucking out Lucas's stall in these boots. Already imagined how they'll look toed into his stirrups. Melinda's wedding is weeks and weeks away. Maybe Em and Lucas will be home for the weekend and I can convince Em to lend me her boyfriend. I'm sure he'd come along for the free dinner if for nothing else.

"I'll take them," I say. Selling my soul to the devil. Or, at least, my sister.

I'm not sure which one's worse.

We stand at the cash and the woman who was helping us pulls out a large bag and starts slotting the items into it.

I watch my beautiful new-to-me boots, and my real-actual breeches disappear into the bag and I have a flashback to my younger self at seven, and eight, and nine – every year of my childhood – being taken to Kiddie Kobbler by my mom to buy a new pair of school shoes. The woman would put the purchase through then wait, and look at my mom who would always say, "She'll wear them home."

We'd leave the store with my old shoes in the new shoe box, and the new shoes on my feet, and it was the best feeling ever.

I want that feeling now. I want to wear those boots out of this store.

But I'm grown-up. I'm sensible. It would just be silly. I'll have lots of chances to wear them.

"Good?" my sister asks. When I hesitate she asks, "What is it?"

I don't know why, but I'm suddenly emboldened to say, "Actually, I think I'd like to wear the boots home."

Rachel grins. "Good for you, sis. Ask for what you want." She glances at her watch. "But you'd better be quick; we need to get back before Melinda starts texting and asking where we are."

Chapter Ten

Melinda isn't happy with the olive boule.

"It has gluten in it," she says when Rachel triumphantly settles the bread on the table.

"Uh, yeah. It's *bread*. Gluten is kind of the point of bread."

"Mmm ... well. I'm not eating gluten until after the wedding."

Beside me Paige shifts in her chair and I watch her spine straighten. She may be the most mild-mannered of my sisters, but push the wrong button, and she's quite possibly the toughest one too. As a medical resident, what she calls "Google Healthcare" is one of her pet peeves. She and my mom didn't speak for a week once when Paige had a cold and my mom gave her a big bottle of **Cold Buster**.

"Just take that the way it says on the bottle, and you'll be fine in a few days," my mom said.

"I'll be fine in a few days anyway, because my immune system will conquer the virus that causes my cold in a few days."

My mom knit her eyebrows. "This stuff really works Paige. I saw an ad on TV for it." We all knew the ad. It featured a certain retired newscaster my mom had adored since her childhood.

"An ad which convinced you to spend nineteen bucks on it. Am I right? You might as well have flushed a twenty-dollar bill down the toilet."

That was the polite part of the conversation. Food fads line up right beside fake medicines in Paige's mind and I know neither of my sisters will back down if this conversation continues.

Right on cue, Paige clears her throat and asks, "Do you even know what gluten is?" while at the exact same time, Rachel holds her hand out and says, "Fine, you can give me twenty bucks for the bread, and another ten for my time."

In the split second of silence that follows, while Melinda decides which of them to take on, I throw myself under the bus.

"I can't find shoes to wear to the wedding!"

Peacekeeper Ellie. Conflict avoider. My sisters call me that like it's a bad thing, but what's so wrong with

everybody just getting along? And my diversion works –
everyone turns to look at me.

Melinda: "What do you mean, you can't find shoes?"

Rachel: "Oh, I'll have to show you the stiletto sandals
I'm wearing ..."

Paige: "I just bought a pair of plain white pumps – they
sell them at the wedding store and they'll dye them to
match ..."

Melinda: "Stilettos? Dyed pumps?"

Shoot. OK, so maybe that wasn't the best peace-mak-
ing topic. I'm racking my brain for something else when
the doorbell rings. "I'll go!"

I don't even have to answer the door, because when I
get into the kitchen I face Lucas, stepping in, calling out,
"Hello!" and the hug I throw around him is both because
I've truly missed him and because surely nobody can
fight about shoes anymore now that Lucas has appeared.

"What are you doing here?" I ask, and my mom's right
behind me, hustling us both back into the dining room,
"Oh my goodness, what a wonderful surprise! Come on
in, sweetheart. I'll find you a chair and you can sit down
with us. Girls, say hi to Lucas."

They mutter in turn, "Lucas," "Lucas," "Lucas," giving
him all the attention they'd give to an annoying little
brother, still eyeing each other up.

My mom's reaching for the extra chair in the corner when Lucas says, "Oh, thanks Mrs. H, but I can't stay. I actually came for Ellie. Although ..." His eyes light on the olive boule. "Is that Primitive Elements bread? 'Cause I'll have a slice of ..." Melinda slaps his outstretched hand.

"Oh no you don't Lucas Fielding. That is mine." Then, while we all watch, she reaches out and takes the exact slice of gluten-filled olive boule Lucas was aiming for. "Pass the butter?" she asks, then doesn't miss a beat as she continues, "Listen we have a lot more things to talk about. We haven't even started on place cards ..."

***

When I excuse myself to follow Lucas to the relative quiet of the kitchen, and he tells me he has tickets to tonight's home-opener, there's no way I need to ask *which* home-opener. My university's basketball team has gone undefeated for three straight years. They're the best team in the country, by far. They often beat visiting teams from the States. Tickets to tonight's season-opening game are near-impossible to come by. "How'd you get those?"

"Our coach is friends with their assistant coach – he got tickets through him," Lucas says. "Coach knows I'm from here – I guess he figured I'd have a place to stay if I came back for the game, so he offered me the tickets."

I lift my eyebrows. "So, it had nothing to do with you winning the free throw challenge in practice last week?"

Lucas's cheeks redden. "Did Em tell you that?"

I nod. "She did. So why didn't you bring her?"

"Oh, you know you're my first choice for watching basketball."

"She has a huge essay due tomorrow, doesn't she?"

He laughs. "That too." He gestures toward the dining room where a quick glance shows Melinda holding court around the table, waving a piece of olive boule as though it's a laser pointer. "So, can you tear yourself away to come with me?"

Rachel comes through the doorway, holding the empty water pitcher.

"I heard," she stage whispers. "Go!"

She thrusts the pitcher under the tap and turns to me. "I wouldn't normally condone you fleeing family conflict – especially when I'm being left behind – but this counts as a social outing, so get yourself out of here – I'll run interference."

***

Lucas's seats are amazing. Front and centre, with nobody blocking our view.

It's a fantastic way to watch the complete and utter blow-out of the game, and it also means when the mascot comes around with t-shirts to throw to the crowd, I actually catch one for the first time in my life.

I pull it on right over the shirt I'm already wearing, and having team colours on makes it even more fun when the team starts pulling away after the first quarter and the gap just widens and widens. First we all wonder, *Can they double the score?*

They do, and the whispers start going around, *Can they pass 100?*

They pull it off with a spectacular dunk from the guy I've seen around campus a few times. He's not their tallest, but is undeniably one of their most consistent players.

Lucas and I jump to our feet, along with the rest of the gym. Even the small contingent of players' families and alumni from the opposing team give polite claps. It was a beautiful basket. It's an impressive score. This team is the kind of powerhouse you don't get to witness very often.

As we're filing out of the bleachers the cheerleaders and several of the players are scattered around the gym floor. People are congratulating them, taking selfies with them. I recognize one or two people from my classes. Lucas sees a few people he knows from basketball. We say hi, exchange a few words, make our way slowly toward the doors.

"Hey man, nice game." I turn and Lucas is talking to dunk guy. Did I say he wasn't one of their tallest players?

That's true, but he's still got a few inches on Lucas. I look way up and smile at him.

His eyes slide to me and Lucas says, "Oh hey, Ellie. This is Terrell. He played with our club team – he was in the age group above Rory and me and he scrimmaged with us – aka wiped the floor with us – a few times. Terrell, this is my neighbour, Ellie. She goes to school here."

The guy puts his hand out. "Hi, Ellie. I actually noticed you in the stands – you were the only one who put your team tee on. Gotta love that team spirit."

I laugh. "If it wasn't for Lucas, you wouldn't have seen me. I normally get stuck in the nosebleeds, but his tickets were fantastic."

"So, you two are neighbours?"

I nod and hip-check Lucas. "Well, and he's dating my best friend."

"Oh yeah?"

Lucas nods. "Yeah. Actually, could we maybe get a selfie with you to send to her? She'd think it was pretty cool."

"Of course. In fact …" Terrell nods into the crowd and a cheerleader appears, and takes Lucas's phone from him.

I hang back. I hate having my photograph taken so much I skipped both of the grad photo days at school last year. It was the one thing that made my normally relaxed mother angry. "Ellie, you are my daughter, I love you, I'm proud of you, and now I don't have a graduation photo of you."

"I'm sorry," I'd said, and meant it – I *was* sorry for her, but I would have been more sorry if there was photographic evidence of how terrible I looked captured forever in the school yearbook.

"Ellie!" Lucas is holding his arm wide.

I shake my head. "You two go ahead."

"Ellie. I did *not* use my extra ticket on you to not have a photo of the occasion."

There are other people waiting for Terrell's attention, and the cheerleader's smile is looking a little forced. I take a deep breath and remember how I looked in the mirror with Rachel the other day, and I slip in between Lucas and Terrell and listen to Rachel's voice saying, *You are so, so pretty.*

I'll settle for not-hideous.

The cheerleader smiles, hands the phone back, and bounces away. Clearly this happens all the time.

I turn back to Terrell. "Thanks for taking the time. It was really nice of you."

"It was my pleasure." It's such a nice thing to say. So much nicer than "no problem," which always makes me think maybe it *was* a little bit of a problem.

"Good to see you again," Lucas says, and I lift a hand in a small wave, and we turn to go, when Terrell clears his throat.

"Actually ..." he says. We stop and I wait for him to ask Lucas something basketball-related, but he looks at me and says. "Since you and Lucas aren't ... well, since you're just neighbours ... well, what I mean is, would you be willing to give me your number?"

I'm struggling to understand. My number? Does he think I'm on the women's basketball team? Does he want to know my jersey number?

I look at Lucas and he lifts his eyebrows and it sinks in. Terrell Campbell, an amazingly good basketball player on this legendary team, wants my phone number. The breath leaves my body.

"I don't know what to say." It's the most honest thing I can think of.

Terrell slaps his forehead. "I'm sorry. I was so hopeful when I heard you weren't Lucas's girlfriend, but that doesn't mean you're single. In fact, I should have known ... someone like you ..."

Someone like me. Wow. He's noticing *me*. Picking *me* out of the sea of people who must be interested in him.

I look at Lucas again because he's my anchor here and he shrugs and leaves me adrift. "It's up to you, Ell."

I have to speak. I have to answer. I lift my gaze to Terrell again. *He does have really kind eyes.* "I'm not ... I mean, I don't ..." I shake my head. "How about this – maybe I could get your number? And I could call you?"

He grins. *Nice white teeth, too.* "I can live with that."

I'm relieved when he holds out his hand for my phone. I'm so flustered I'd forget how to enter a new contact, and I'd probably scramble the numbers.

When he hands it back, I say, "OK, great then. Thanks for doing that," and he says. "I hope you decide to call," and I say, "Yeah. OK," and I feel sorry for him if he's trying to read my intentions because I don't have the slightest idea what I plan to do.

As Lucas and I walk out of the gym he leans over and says, "So, *that* just happened."

Yeah. I guess it did.

***

In the train on the way home Lucas shows me the photo the cheerleader took. "It's good," he says.

"It is." There's something I really like about Terrell's eyebrows. I'm not about to tell Lucas that, though. I zoom in and, sure enough, there it is, an ever-so-faint scar above his lip that I noticed while we were talking. It's a tiny imperfection that makes him that much more perfect.

Also, I look ... fine. OK, maybe better than fine. My hair is shiny, and so are my eyes, and my skin isn't, and my smile looks genuine.

It's the nicest picture I've seen of myself in years.

I hand the phone back to Lucas and he thumbs around a bit and says, "There, I sent it to you and Em."

"Good. She'll like it."

"You could send it to Terrell. I mean, you have his number."

I snort. "I'm pretty sure he wouldn't want it."

"I'm pretty sure he might." He snaps his fingers. "You know who I should send it to ..."

And I do. From the set of his jaw, and the steel in his voice, I can tell right away.

"No," I say. "Please don't."

"He should see how well you're doing. He should see ..."

"Lucas, I appreciate your support, but what happened between Rory and me – it sucks that it ruined your friendship."

"He hurt you, Ellie. That's not OK."

Lucas is right. He did. But after talking to Addy and Rachel, after hearing what Rachel said, it's amazing how much of the hurt is gone. Maybe Rachel's right, and Rory was dealing with his own issues. Or maybe not, but does it really matter?

"You know what, Lucas, it did hurt a lot at first, but I'm OK now."

"I should still send it ..."

"I'll make you a deal. I'll send the photo to Terrell if you promise not to send it to Rory."

Lucas tilts his head. "Really? That's not a move I'd expect from you. Although, don't get me wrong, I totally approve."

I select Terrell's newly entered name from my contacts, find the photo, and thumb a quick message **Thanks again for the photo. A good way to remember a great game.** I send it and hold it up for Lucas. "See? Gone."

He grins. "Well played, Ms. Hannaman. On both counts."

As I slip my phone back in my pocket I hope he's right.

Chapter Eleven

Saturday morning my mom catches me reading up on Terrell.

It starts innocently enough – reading Dr. Hamilton's latest newsletter – this one about a former patient who just made it into vet school. She's pictured holding a beagle, beaming. It would be hard to say which one of the two is cuter.

Vet school. That could be fun. I might not exactly have the right prerequisites just yet, but I could look into it.

That makes me think of school.

I click to our school site. Skip the "sciences" tab to click on "athletics." From there the trip to **basketball → men's → bios →** and **Terrell Campbell**, just seems like a natural flow.

Each player has a profile page and Terrell's mentions he's a hometown player. Quotes him that one of his weak points is not always being mean enough on the court. Cites his former coach calling him an example on and off the court, saying, "He's just an all-around nice person."

Awww ...

Which is when my mom sticks her head around the door, and I fumble for the home button, and my wrist teeter-totters the glass of orange juice by my side.

"Everything OK?" my mom asks.

"Oh, yeah. Fine."

"What are you looking at?"

My mom and I don't really fight. I'm really lucky to have a mother who's there for me while also respecting my privacy. She's always understanding. Given all these things I should probably just tell her the truth. That I met Terrell. That I might, possibly, maybe be interested in him.

But ... even if she's a great one, she's still my *mom*. I don't really want to go into details of my love life with her.

So, I do the obvious thing. I snap at her. "Nothing, OK? What is this? The Spanish Inquisition?"

My mom blinks. Bites her lip. "I'm sorry. I didn't mean it as an inquisition. I was just interested."

Guilt. Instant and all-encompassing. She never pried about Rory. When I told her we broke up, she just said, "I'm really, really sorry," and baked me an apple pie. One I didn't have to share with my sisters. It's not my mother's fault I'm self-conscious about my relationships.

"No, I'm the one who's sorry." I stand, close my laptop, and drain the last of my juice. "I shouldn't have talked to you that way. I must be stressed."

My mom holds her hand out for my empty glass. "Don't worry about it, Ellie. You have a lot going on. All the more reason for you to get out to the barn and have a little break this morning."

"Thanks, Mom."

I won't snap at her again, I tell myself, and feel the guilt begins to ebb away, replaced by excitement about wearing my new-to-me riding boots.

***

My laptop-exchange with my mom means I'm early again, but this time I don't just sit in the car. I head straight to Lucas's barn.

At first, I'm disappointed to find it's empty but then I notice the unoccupied stalls are dirty and it just takes a slow walk around the small barn for me to find a pitchfork hung on the wall above the wheelbarrow.

I know what to do next.

Is it weird to enjoy sifting, and lifting, and tossing manure and dirty shavings? Because I do enjoy it. I make it through Oreo's stall in no time and, hardly breaking my rhythm, I cross the aisle to Lucas's.

Lift-shake-heave-fluff, lift-shake-heave-fluff ... I work my way around Lucas's stall too, and now both have banks of clean, light shavings around the walls and bare expanses of rubber matting in the centre.

There's a whistle from the doorway, and I turn to see Sasha. "These stalls look amazing!" she says. "What a great job!"

"Oh, thanks. I probably did something wrong ..."

She's shaking her head. "You know, there's not really much you can do *wrong* about cleaning a stall. Especially when it means somebody else doesn't need to clean it."

"Now," she says. "Do you want me to help you finish in here, then I'll help you bring Lucas in?"

Finishing up involves washing out water buckets and sweeping the small aisle between the two stalls. "I like to do this other stuff before I put the clean bedding in," Sasha explains. "That way the rubber matting can really dry out."

Sure enough, a couple of large spots that were initially darker than the rest of the matting are now shrinking away to nothing.

Once there's a nice layer of fresh wood-smelling shavings in both stalls, Sasha says, "Grab a lead rope and we'll go get Lucas."

**

The main sound as we stride across the stableyard is the crunch of gravel under our boots ... *my nice new boots* ... as if she's reading my mind, Sasha stops and points, "Hey! Nice boots!"

"Thank you."

"Are they comfortable?"

I nod.

"Well then you'll have them forever."

Forever. It doesn't seem like something a twelve-year-old would say, but maybe she's heard it from her mom. Also, clearly, Sasha is not a normal twelve-year-old.

Whatever – it has a nice ring to it. I'll have them forever. That means I'll be riding forever ... right?

"There he is." Sasha lifts her hand toward a paddock ahead of us and, sure enough, there's a familiar brown horse, head down, flanked by two other brown horses.

Sasha's busy explaining, "Normally he goes out with the herd," – along with her own adorable pony, Oreo – "... but the two he's with here are new, and Laney wanted to turn them out with a reliable horse, and that's Lucas ..."

I'm half listening, but I'm also noticing how Lucas's head has lifted and how his ears are pitched forward, and how he's ambling, slowly and surely, toward the gate.

"He's coming for you!" Sasha says. "That says a lot when there's still hay left!"

"He isn't really, is he?" My heart does a funny hiccupping thing – like its beat has been interrupted – in a good way.

Lucas has his head over the gate now, nostrils flared, and he snorts wide and wet when we get up to him. Sasha ducks and lets me take the brunt of the spray. "Yup. I'd say that's for you! Since Em's not here, you're his *person.*"

"Oh!" I'm swamped with an uprush of emotion. I know I'm surrounded by people who love me, but while Em has Lucas, and Melinda has Bill, and my parents have each other – and four daughters – I don't feel like I've ever been anyone's particularly special person. Now, this horse – he's chosen *me.*

"Hi Bud," I say, and he bumps my outstretched hand with his muzzle, and I feel the most confident I've felt so far since starting this whole riding journey.

Because surely, surely, if I can learn Calculus, like I did last year, and write essays on Beowulf, then I can also learn the minute details of horse care, and I've already got the big thing – the thing you can't learn or force – I've got the love and trust of this animal.

It's pretty cool.

***

Rising trot is possibly harder than Calculus.

Holy hell. How is anyone supposed to do this? And how long will Lucas keep loving me while I'm slamming down on his back like this?

Because that's what this is – not rising trot, but slamming, bouncing, jostling trot.

"You just have to relax!" I'm not sure whether to be flattered that Laney seems to trust me enough to leave me under Sasha's supervision while she focuses on the much-younger riders, or to be mortified that a twelve-year-old is my teacher.

Whatever way I slice it, Sasha knows way more than I do, so she's the boss.

"C-c-a-n we w-w-alk?" I manage to ask over a long series of teeth-rattling jounces.

"Sure! Walk Lucas." Lucas has already gotten the message, and drops to his walk, which I now recognize as being smooth-as-glass.

I sigh, blow upward, forgetting I'm wearing a helmet so there's no hair to move off my forehead. "OK, I get the *idea* of relaxing – I understand why it would work – but there's no way I can relax when I'm bouncing around like that."

Sasha nods. "Gotcha. Let's try something different."

"Whoa! Whoa! Whoa!" We're both distracted by Laney yelling from the other end of the ring. A pony rams its nose up another pony's bum, and I guess they must be friends because nothing bad happens.

Laney strides over to yank Pony Number Two's nose away from Pony Number One's backside, and I turn my concentration back to Sasha. "Sorry," I say.

"No," Sasha says. "It's OK. Actually, it's good. I think you're relaxed."

"Oh, I guess maybe I am."

She bounces on her toes. "Let's use that. Here's what you should do. Breathe, now."

I breathe. Deeply.

"How does that feel?"

"Good."

"So you just need to keep feeling that way."

"How do I do that?"

Sasha shrugs. "Well, we can ask Laney if you like, but I'd say, just keep breathing."

I breathe again, and beneath me Lucas gives a long, rattling exhale.

"Oh!" Sasha claps several times. "Now you exhale too!"

"What?"

"Exhale! Like him! Rattling your lips."

"I ..." *Oh, whatever.* I exhale and let my lips go loose, and as I do it Lucas lowers his head and his strides come long and swingier.

"Ask him to trot," Sasha says. "But *gently* and *keep breathing!*"

I have no idea if I can do this, but I guess it's worth trying.

I remember what Sasha told me the first time we tried trotting. I push my hands into Lucas's mane and squeeze the muscles all along my legs. And – oh yeah – I keep breathing.

The lurch from the walk – which I've totally mastered (or at least I feel like I have) – to the terrifying, jaw-clenching, bone-shaking trot, actually comes as less of a jolt this time and more of a spring.

My relaxed hips bounce forward, then they fall back.

"I am?"

"Yes. Just let him push you up, then settle back down, then up again ... just the way you're doing."

"But this is easy. This is no work at all."

Sasha smacks her forehead. "That's the idea. It's not supposed to be hard. You're not supposed to fight him."

"You're posting!" Laney's walked over from the other end of the ring where the little kids are standing in a more-or-less neat row with their ponies being held by their parents. Laney saying it makes me totally believe it; I *must* have been posting.

All of a sudden the trot is smooth, easy, flowing. I can't figure out what I had against it before.

I can see now that Lucas's trot is the equivalent of my half-marathon run pace; steady, rhythmic – something I can sustain all day.

"I love it!" I say.

"Good job," says Laney. "To both of you. Maybe just work on it both directions, then do some walk-trot transitions, and that will be good for today."

"Thanks," I say. And my thanks is for Laney, and Sasha, and Lucas, and Em.

***

Sasha's showing me how to clean tack. This, like the stall mucking, is surprisingly satisfying. There's something about watching the leather come up dark, and clean, with just a light sheen, under my circling cloth.

"That's good," Sasha's telling me. "Lots of people use too much saddle soap. You're not trying to make *suds*." She says "suds" like it's one of *those* four-letter words. "You're a natural."

"Hmm ... I wish I could stay and do this all day, because I'm definitely not a natural at trying on fancy clothes, which is what I have to do this afternoon."

"Oh? Why?" Sasha reaches across, showing me how to use the edge of my fingernail to gently lift a dark spot of grime off the leather.

"My sister's wedding's coming up and I'm a bridesmaid. She's chosen ugly dresses that don't look very comfortable, either. We have a fitting this afternoon."

"Lu-cky ..." Sasha breathes.

I tilt my head and wrinkle my nose. "You don't strike me as the fussy dress type."

"Oh no ... not that part ... it's just I've never been to a wedding."

I lift my eyebrows. "Well, take it from me, it's not as exciting as you think. And there's pretty much no escaping wearing a dress, so ..."

Sasha sighs. "Yeah, you're probably right. Anyway, I'm sure I'll get to go to one someday." She brushes her hands together. "You're done! That bridle looks really good. I'll show you how to buckle it into a figure-eight when you hang it up."

***

From the car I can see Sasha lead her pony out to the sand ring. She mounts up and I know what that feels like.

She rides in a wide, slow, easy loop around the track, and I can imagine doing that, too.

Eventually she moves into a trot, and begins rising effortlessly, and pride swells in me because sure, I know how it feels to do that wrong, but now I also know how it feels to do it right.

I take out my phone and text Em **Great news!**

You're in love! she replies.

You know it.

Let me guess, it's his big brown eyes.

Oh yes. And the way he nuzzles my neck.

And his perfect backside.

With those long, lean legs. All four of them ...

I knew you'd fall for him ... now tell me your great news.

Learned to do rising trot. Probably not a big deal.

A HUGE deal! It's not easy. So proud of you!

I smile as I turn the key in the ignition. I've been taught not to brag, but the truth is I'm kind of proud of myself, too.

Chapter Twelve

Indian Summer. That's what they call days like this as Fall is in full, spectacular bloom, when the maples are fiery, geese honk their way in waving vees through the searing blue sky, and the sun burns strong enough that when I close my eyes and turn to face it, I can see orange on the inside of my eyelids.

It's the time of year for ornaments made of dried corn, and potted chrysanthemums in their muted autumn colours, and pumpkins on front porches.

"Indian Summer ..." My mom pauses from unloading the dishwasher to gaze out the window. She turns to me and asks, "Is it still OK to call it that?"

Good question. "I don't know, Mom. I mean, it's something nice, so I hope it's OK."

"Maybe I'll try to find out today." My mom works in the local library as a library assistant which means she mostly reshelves books and, every two weeks changes the displays on the bulletin boards. She loves her job and reveres the librarians she assists. If anyone will find out about the political correctness of Indian Summer, it's my mom.

I love her for her awareness, and sensitivity, and curiosity, but I'm not brave enough to tell her so. Instead I say, "Make sure you tell me when you find out."

"OK." She stretches onto her tiptoes to kiss me on the cheek. "I love you too, honey."

***

Indian Summer, or not, today feels like a good day. I like the classes I have. I get back my first short essay with an eighty-four per cent scrawled on it. I've always heard people who pull off good grades at high school are in for a shock at university – when the best and the brightest all come together and it becomes much harder to shine. But eighty-four per cent is a decent mark, and the prof's provided notes. I feel like if I read them through maybe I can get eighty-six next time.

At lunch I find a rock that's been sun-bathed all morning, soaking up warmth. When I sit on it, the heat radiates through the fabric of my jeans. I stretch my legs in front of me and admire my new-to-me boots – Rachel was right; they're good for more than just riding. I can hardly believe those are my feet – they must surely be the feet of a cooler, wealthier, more stylish person.

My leftover pearl-barley-and-chickpea salad tastes even better than when I made it yesterday, and even when a breeze cold enough to ripple goosebumps across my skin whirls in from the river bordering the campus,

I'm OK with it. After all, if it was too warm I'd just look silly wearing leather boots.

Which your sister will take back from you if you don't invite someone to Melinda's wedding.

Even that little doomsday voice can't bother me today. On a day like this, anything seems possible. I'll see Addy in class this afternoon and our budding friendship will continue to grow. I don't want to jinx this thing with Terrell but the fact that he replied to my photo text with **Nice!!!** means it's not impossible I'll have a date for the wedding.

I'll keep the boots. Everything will be OK.

***

Addy's late for class. I only realize how much I was looking forward to seeing her when the prof starts talking, and the seat next to me is still empty.

I haven't known her for that long, but despite the crazy amount of activities she does, I've never known her to be late. I wonder if something's wrong – if she's sick – I pull out my phone to send a surreptitious text when she appears in the doorway.

Our eyes meet and I tap the seat next to me, pull my books toward my side of the table. She tiptoes across the front of the class, head down, muttering, "'Scuse me, pardon me, sorry ..."

She drops into her seat and I try to catch her eye, to smile at her, to lift an eyebrow in a *"Hey, what's up – everything OK?"* kind of way.

She dodges me, though. Head down, leafing through her notes. One hand pulling her turtleneck up high. A sideways whisper. "Talk to you at break."

I know the signs. I've been there, felt that. Had every good intention to leave the house on time then took one, last, fatal look in the mirror. Saw a blemish staring back at me that made it obvious, there was no way I could go out in public like that.

Except, the results of attacking it were almost always worse.

Sure enough, later in class, as Addy's guard, and her turtleneck drop, I get a glimpse of a large, angry red welt on her jawline. *I'm sorry,* I want to tell her. *I understand. It sucks.*

I know hearing those things right now would not be helpful, though. You can only obsess about your skin for so long – sometimes distraction is the best option. So when the prof tells us all to take a five-minute break, I say, "Do you understand all the conditions for invoking the Notwithstanding Clause, because I think I'm a little mixed up ..."

And she says, "What part's confusing you?" And we both use our brains, and think hard, and I hope that helps. I'm not positive, though, because as our in-depth conversation ends, and the prof starts scribbling on the board again, Addy pulls up the neck of her shirt and sinks her chin down into it.

At the end of class, Addy and I start walking toward the bike racks like we always do. She squints up at the sky. "Too bad it's so beautiful – I was kind of hoping you wouldn't have your bike today."

"Why?"

"A couple of girls on my floor are in the other Legal Studies section and they have the same assignment as us. We were going to have a study group meeting tonight. I was hoping you could come, but I guess you can't ride your bike home after dark."

For the last while I've avoided meeting new people. It was never easy. I didn't know if they were really staring at me, or I was just imagining they were. Either way, I could never relax enough to be light-hearted, fun, good company. Not like Addy does. It's one of the things I really admire about her.

I want to make her happy. Want to grow our friendship. "We-e-ell ..."

"What?" she asks.

"If I take the train, I can bring my bike on it."

"Yeah? How close does that get you to home?"

"My mom would probably pick me up from the station if I texted her." I'm still thinking this through. Still uncertain.

Addy, though, is full speed ahead. "I bet she'd come here to get you. It wouldn't be 'till later. Way after rush hour. I can show you my room, and you can join us for dinner at the caf. Then we're going to study at these secret tables one of the girls found. Tucked around the corner from Tim Horton's and – more importantly – the women's washroom, with great scenery."

"Won't it be dark?" I ask.

She laughs. "You'll see what I mean."

***

Because she won a scholarship, Addy has a room to herself. It's compact, but it feels airy thanks to the white-painted breezeblock walls, and the sunset flooding in through the west-facing windows.

"Nice view!" I stand so close to the glass I can feel the cold of the quickly dropping temperature outside. My eye travels across grass and trees to the sparkle of tiny waves on the canal in the distance.

Addy nods. "It's not home, but I can't really complain."

"Speaking of home, is that it?" I cross to a collage of photos held in place by criss-crossed webbing on a board over her desk.

There's a picture of a house that's nothing special – not new, but not old, clad in a non-descript beigey tone – but behind it is an expanse of water with no limits that I can see. "The Ottawa River?" I ask.

"Yep."

"So, yeah, I can see why the canal maybe doesn't quite cut it."

She laughs. "I can't complain. I really wasn't sure about living in the city, but as cities go, this one's pretty manageable."

There are lots of family photos, too. A black-and-tan dog features in many of them. "I'm a sucker for dogs like that," I say.

"Mutts?"

"If that's what he is, then yes."

Except for one picture, which shows a man in a plaid shirt with a baseball cap turned backward, the rest of the photos showcase various combinations of a curly-haired woman who looks tiny but strong, Addy, and another girl – always with a beaming smile – sitting in a high-backed wheelchair.

Addy steps forward. "That's my dad. He's in Alberta. The story is he works there because the pay's so good and he can send lots of money home. The truth is, I don't think he knows how to deal with Bethany." She taps a photo. "My sister. She has cerebral palsy."

She shrugs. "Or, who knows? Maybe it's me he can't deal with. Or my mom, who basically all she ever does is deal with Bethany."

"Does she always smile like that, or is she just way better than me when a camera's pointed at her?" I ask.

Addy's quiet for a minute. When I turn she's blinking. "Sorry," she says. "You asking that – it reminds me that she does smile most of the time. She's amazing. I miss her."

I squeeze her arm. "Hey. Of course you do." I point at the board. "I'd miss all that if I had to leave it behind, too."

Addy's stomach gives a huge growl and she laughs. "Ha! So much for emotions. My stomach doesn't care. Do you want to go eat?"

***

We meet her friends at the caf. They're named Olivia and Sophia and they come from the same small town just outside Kingston. They take it upon themselves to educate me in the ways of the cafeteria.

"It was pretty exciting on Day One, wasn't it, Liv?" Sophia asks.

Sophia nods. "Yeah. A huge salad bar and serve-yourself ice cream."

Olivia jumps in again. "But it didn't take long for the salad bar to get down to iceberg lettuce, stale croutons, facon bits, and some extra-lumpy Thousand Island dressing ..."

"... and the only ice cream flavours left are vanilla and tiger tail," Sophia finishes.

All I can say is "facon bits?"

"Mmm ..." Olivia says. "You know, fake bacon. Which, did you know, is vegan?"

"No ..." my voice trails off. These girls make me feel like there's quite a lot I don't know, but they seem happy to teach me, so I obediently follow when they say, "OK, here's what you need to start with ..."

***

Turns out the secret tables Addy mentioned are in a quiet corner of the Athletic Centre and the scenery she talked about isn't whatever's behind the now-pitch-black floor-to-ceiling windows behind us, but rather the parade of varsity athletes going by.

Sophia has a crush on one of the hockey players and I'm not sure how much work she's getting done as she pretends not to be looking for him every five minutes.

When a group of guys drop enormous hockey bags by the wall opposite us, and disappear around the corner Sophia says, "Oh my God. They're going to Tim Horton's. They always go after practice. Someone has to go stand in line behind them right now."

"Why?" Addy asks.

"To hear what they say. They might talk about him. They might mention if he has a girlfriend."

Addy gives me a double-raised-eyebrow look. "Why don't you go?" she asks Sophia.

"Um, obviously because first, I can't let them see me, and second, since he doesn't seem to be with them right now, I need to stay here in case he walks by."

Addy's eyebrows lift even higher, and Olivia opens her mouth to chime in, and I say. "You know what? I need to stretch anyway, so quick – put in your orders and I'll go."

"You're too nice," Addy tells me.

I shrug.

"His name's Eddie," Sophia says.

"How about a box of assorted Timbits?" I ask.

"Yes, good ..." Sophia shoves a twenty-dollar bill in my hand. "Go!"

Sophia was right. I round the corner to find half-a-dozen big, sweaty guys lined up for coffee in front of me. They aren't talking about anyone named Eddie, or whether he has a girlfriend, or about girls at all. They mostly seem to be talking about how bad one another's hockey equipment smells, and asking each other when the last time they each had a shower was.

Which doesn't make me want to stand too close to them.

I let them step forward, and I hang back and decide I'll pay attention if I hear the name "Eddie" but, other than that it's time to make the important decision about whether to let the girl behind the counter give me assorted Timbits or to proactively intervene to avoid having a majority of old-fashioned plain.

Because my brain has prioritized any mention of Eddie, followed by Timbit flavours, it takes me a minute to register someone clearing their throat behind me. Quite loudly. I whirl around to face Terrell and go instantly hot from my toes to my cheeks. My very, very hot cheeks.

"Hi," he says.

"Hi."

Speaking of hot, he looks it. No, that's wrong, he doesn't *look* hot – he *is* hot. I have this overwhelming urge to touch him. Any part of him. Make a stupid excuse by plucking lint off his sleeve, or straightening ... something ... but he's wearing warm ups in the kind of stretchy athletic fabric that doesn't gather lint, and is meant to be slouchy so I keep my hands to myself while my blushing face flames on.

"Come here often?"

"Um, no. I mean, I usually run in the morning before class. At home. I'm not on any teams. I'm actually just here to study ..." He's winking. Why is he winking? *Oh, it's a joke.* I didn't know my cheeks could get hotter, but they do. I semi-rally. "I'm only here for the baked goods."

"Terr ..." the voice is coming from further down the hall, toward the gym. It's followed by "... rell ..." and then a third calls, "Trell!"

I take advantage of his momentary distraction to step sideways, out from under a potlight shining directly down on me. Nobody's skin looks perfect under a spotlight. Although, having said that, Terrell's is invitingly smooth. "Your admiring public?" I ask him.

"My annoying teammates."

They're still hooting and hollering his name. I'm afraid if they keep it up long enough, one of my study group will hear and come over to see what all the noise is about. "You'd better go," I say.

"I don't have any," he says.

"Any what?"

"Admirers."

"I don't feel like that can be true."

He shrugs. Gives his head a sideways tilt. "I guess maybe it depends on who's doing the admiring."

Oh, wow. The truth is, right here, right now, I do, so, admire him. I'd like a chance to admire him more. The ball is definitely in my court. I took his number. I haven't done anything with it, other than send the photo. If I don't do something any chance of any admiring might be gone forever.

I want to be brave. Want to be like Addy, who can talk to anyone, anytime. Or Rachel, who can seduce any guy, anytime. But I'm not them. I'm me. Which means maybe I should just be me ... "I was wondering ... I mean, would you consider ... do you run?"

"Run?"

"Yeah. You know, like to train for basketball."

He nods. "Sure. Yeah."

"Well do you think we could maybe run together?"

He blinks a couple of times. Wrinkles his nose. Lifts a hand and rubs his forehead.

It seems like a reasonable compromise to me. Time spent together, without the pressure of a date. Fine, right? Or maybe that's the problem – it's not fine. It's weird. He's back-pedaling on liking me.

"I'd love to."

"Really?"

"Nothing I'd rather do."

"I thought you were going to say no."

He grins and his teeth shine, eyes sparkle, with just that tiny scar to remind me he's not completely flawless – he's just a human being like me. Or, sort of ... "I was wondering if I'll be able to keep up with you."

"Ha!" It bursts out of me short and sharp, and before I can think I'm standing next to him, pressing my leg to his, saying, "Excuse me – but if you can't keep up to me with legs that long, your coach should be kicking you off the team."

"Maybe that's what I'm afraid of," he says.

And that's when I realize I'm touching him, and the last time I touched a guy was when Rory pulled away as though I'd burned him, and I'm hit with a one-two combo of sadness and hope.

Hope, I decide. *Focus on the hope*, and the decision rockets a fizz of happiness through me. I'm going to run, which is one of my favourite things. With this guy, who I might not really know yet, but who looks great, and seems nice and, most importantly, who seems to like me.

"Well, great," I say. "It'll be fun."

"When?" he asks.

"Sunday?" I suggest. "I think I can do that if my sister doesn't stick in a last-minute wedding planning activity."

"Sunday should be OK for me as long as coach doesn't throw in a last-minute practice."

"So, you check and I'll check and we'll touch base before Sunday?"

He steps forward and leans in, and he's really quite close, and for a second I wonder, *Is he going to kiss me?* He pauses, and winks and says, "Deal."

I watch him walking away with my hand pressed to my cheek and for the first time I can remember it's not covering the spot where I wish nobody would look; it's marking the place where I wish his lips had landed.

Wow.

I turn back to face the counter to find not a single hockey player in sight. *Whoops.* I guess the least I can do is get the Timbits.

To make up for getting no information at all about Eddie, I tell the girl I want lots and lots of chocolate glazed and watch her like a hawk to make sure every second Timbit she picks is chocolate, then I head back to the table with my peace offering.

* * *

Addy's standing with me in the heated area between the double doors of the Athletic Centre while we wait for my mom to pull up in front.

"Do you think you'll take the Social Justice and Human Rights course next year?" I ask.

"I think so …" Her hand strays to her chin. "I've heard good things about the professor .. *shit!*"

"What?"

"I did it again." She pulls her hand away to reveal a welling spot of blood. "I am so stupid."

I fish in my bag. "Don't be silly. Here." I hold out a tissue. "I always have them with me. Habit. Although lately

I've had to also start carrying around lip balm, and eye drops, and moisturizer." I shake my head. "If I don't stay on top of it, the Acnegon makes everything so dry."

Addy blots the blood away. "Are the side effects really as terrible as everyone says?"

I know what she means. My stomach churned with nerves the first time I took a pill. I'd heard it called the "scorched earth approach" to acne control. Some people called it the "nuclear option."

"I think it's different for everyone," I tell her. "Thank goodness, I haven't really had any joint pain. The dryness is real, though. I finally had to give in and put Vaseline up my nose to stop the nosebleeds. But it also took quite a while to work for me. Maybe if it had worked sooner, I'd have had worse side effects? I don't know."

I blink. Flashback to just a couple of months ago when it seemed even the nuclear option wasn't helping me and I thought, *if not this, then what?* I'd called in sick to work for the first time ever, and called Rachel to take me to an emergency appointment with Dr. Hamilton.

"It's hard, I know." Dr Hamilton had said. "You're doing all the right things. I believe it will work. But I'm glad you came to see me."

She was right. It was amazing how suddenly my skin had cleared up. Which is probably why I still couldn't quite believe it. Why a voice in my head I tried not to listen to kept telling me it could all come back just as quickly.

I shake my head. *Focus on Addy.* "Is it the side effects that keep you from using it?"

She sighs. "No. I mean, don't get me wrong, they make me nervous. But ..." She bites her lip. "I hope this doesn't offend you ..."

"I won't be offended. I promise."

"Well, with my sister's medical challenges, this just seemed silly. Unimportant. Cosmetic. Between all Bethany's appointments for really, truly serious issues, I'm sure it would never have crossed my mom's mind to take me to a doctor for acne."

"I get it, Addy. To be honest, I'm glad now that my skin's cleared up, but I also almost feel like I cheated. Like I don't deserve it, especially when I think of the things other people are going through."

"Of course you do," she says.

I look her straight in the eye. "Maybe you do too, then?"

She drops my gaze. "I don't know ... I'm not in high school anymore. It shouldn't be that big a deal."

"But it is. You know that. I mean, sure, it's not cancer, or cerebral palsy, but it hurts, and it makes life hard. It's worth fixing."

"Yeah, well, I wouldn't even know how to begin. There aren't exactly a lot of dermatologists in a town of 2,500 people."

"They have them here, though. My sister helped me. I could help you."

She lifts her hand. "It's OK. It's not your problem. And, anyway I'm thinking your mom's here."

"How do you know?"

She points at a car that's just pulled up to the curb outside. Inside is my mom, waving frantically, smiling ear-to-ear. "Either that woman is very disturbed, or she's very happy to see you."

"My mom really does love her girls," I say.

"Go," she says. "Don't keep her waiting."

"But ..."

"But nothing. We talked. It was good. We'll talk again some other time."

"Any time," I say.

She nods. "OK, any time."

Chapter Thirteen

I blink at my bedside clock.

It's Saturday, right? Yes, definitely Saturday. I shouldn't be awake this early.

In fact, I very much resent being awake this early, because I was deeply cocooned in a dream that felt very real, where Terrell was just about to give me that kiss I'd been waiting for back at Tim Horton's.

And then, intrusion. Something. What was it? Dragging me from sleep. Pulling me into unwilling semi-consciousness.

There is it again. Melinda's voice.

Another squint at the clock. What is she doing here so early?

Crying.

When I shuffle into the kitchen, yawning, and stretching, and using my fingers to work sleep tangles out of my hair, Melinda's sitting at the table, with my mom sitting next to her, and her eyes and nose are red, and she's sniffing.

"Morning?" I venture, because it's clearly not a good morning for Melinda.

"Good morning honey," my mom says. "You sit here with your sister and I'll make you both pancakes."

I wait for Melinda to protest the gluten, or the butter, or the maple syrup, but maybe, like me, the comfort she associates with sitting at my mom's table, being fed pancakes is too huge to ever turn them down.

While my mom measures, and mixes, and pours, and flips, I turn to Melinda. "So, um, is everything OK?"

Sniff-sniff. "Everything sucks."

"Oh." I spin the maple syrup bottle one way, then the other. "Do you want to talk about it?"

"No." I'm about to say, 'OK' when she continues. "No. It stresses me out to even think about it. I mean, there's still so much to do, and nobody takes it as seriously as me. Bill wanted red velvet cake and I saw a sample last night and it's *horrible*. Terrible. But it's the one thing he wants, so I can't say no. But the one thing I want is for him to care as much as I do, and he just doesn't." She pauses for a shaky breath.

"He doesn't worry about anything, and he doesn't tell me things. The dress arrived last night for his niece – the one who was going to be the lead flower girl and corral all the other little tiny flower girls – and that's when he told me she wasn't coming. He *forgot* that she got accepted as a boarder at the National Ballet School. How do you forget that? And when was he going to tell me? And when I said it would be a disaster to have all the really small girls in the ceremony without his niece to guide them, he said maybe we just wouldn't be able to have any flower girls. Which ... no flower girls, Ellie? I mean ..." She lifts her hands, then lets them fall in the classic, *Words fail* gesture. *Mmm ... salty butter, and sweet syrup, and fluffy pancakes ...*

My mom slides a plate of pancakes in front of each of us, and I mumble, "Thanks Mom," and drown mine in a lake of syrup, and take a bite.

My brain perks up. The gears start grinding.

I turn to Melinda. "How old is Bill's niece?"

The carbs and sugar have chased some of the desperation out of her eyes. In fact, she looks mostly puzzled. "Huh? What? Twelve, but why do you care?"

I swallow a bite of pancake. "If you trust me, I think I might be able to solve your flower girl problem."

She chews and swallows. Takes a sip of coffee. Sets her cup down and says, "I suppose I'm going to have to. Don't make me regret it." Then she turns to my mom. "Thanks, Mom. I'm feeling a lot more like myself."

No kidding.

✳✳✳

My car is always the first one in the stable parking lot on Saturday mornings.

Or, so far it always has been.

Today there's a substantial pick-up truck in the yard. The mud-encrusted, lug-tired truck has a trailer coupled to it stacked with a wall of hay.

It's blocking where I normally park, so I slow to a crawl and pick a spot as far away from the truck as possible, pulling in, then sitting and wondering what to do.

Rap-rap-rap ... sharp knuckles striking my passenger window, followed by Sasha's grinning face not more than an inch from the glass, and her voice, muffled by the glass, saying, "You've come at just the right time!"

It's amazing how much being wanted can lift your heart. With a smile stretching my cheeks, I swing my door open to face Sasha, who's already run around to my side of the car. "So, tell me – why is this just the right time?"

***

Because there's hay to unload.

"Just a bit," Sasha said. This family down the road, she explained, just sold their daughter's horse. Which left them with a barn stocked with hay for the winter, and no horse to eat it.

"They're offering a good price, and there's room in the loft, so Laney told them to bring it over."

"What do you need me to do?" I ask.

"Come on up with me!"

Since Lucas is in the smaller barn, I don't spend much time in the main barn, and I guess I never really noticed the ladder to nowhere.

Of course, as soon as I follow Sasha up the steep set of rungs nailed to the wall, I realize they don't go nowhere at all. The slight girl disappears into the darkness above, and when I reach the disappearing point it's like climbing through a vertical tunnel.

There are bales stacked on the floor all around the square opening. They block the light, muffle sounds. It reminds me of the sound absorbing Quiet Cube at the Science Museum.

I pause for a second, and the absence of noise around me creates its own sound – a kind of rush that's probably my own blood rushing around my head, but seems like it could also be the voice of the cosmos. Or something like that ...

"Ellie! Hurry!" Silence doesn't last long with Sasha around.

I've only seen haylofts a couple of times on TV or in movies, where they look like magical places washed with golden-warm light and full of straw heaped in soft piles, where cute girls with perfect waves in their hair cavort with hot guys wearing jeans that fit just right.

Don't get me wrong – the hay loft is neat – I like it. But the first activity that comes to mind when I gaze around the quite cold, fairly dim, and definitely dusty space is hide-and-seek.

This is a place for climbing, and darting, and contorting oneself behind tightly packed bales. I rest my hand on one of those bales long enough to confirm, yup, it's just as scratchy as it looks. There's no way a romantic rendezvous up here could end in anything but an angry rash and underpants full of hay.

Turns out it's not just erotic romps that will rough your skin and work chaff into undergarments – by the time I'm done grabbing hay bales off the clunking, clicking, grinding conveyor belt and slinging them in Laney's direction, for her to stack properly, not only are my arms aching but I feel like the scarecrow from the Wizard of Oz.

Unloading hay is hard work, and the hay dust mixed with the sweat on my forehead is probably not the kind of facial mask beauty sites recommend.

When Sasha and I climb back to the bottom of the ladder, I thrust my hand into my breeches pocket. Oh yeah ... I'm going to have to turn all my pockets inside-out before I put any of these clothes in the washing machine. As for my underwear ... "Is there somewhere I can change?" I ask Sasha.

"Huh? You're already wearing your riding clothes."

"Well, not *change*, exactly. More like peel my clothes off and shake them out so I don't get a rash when I ride."

She giggles. "That's why I wear a belt – *tight* – with my t-shirt tucked in."

"You could have told me!"

She shrugs. "Some things you just have to learn for yourself, Rookie! Anyway, in Lucas's stall."

"In Lucas's stall, what?"

"That's where you should change, of course. It's private, and you can't exactly go inside anywhere to shake half-a-ton of hay all over the floor, can you?"

"Really? Change in a stall?"

We're already walking toward the small barn and she turns and throws a wink over her shoulder. "I'll tell you a secret. In January a stall is warmer than using the port-a-potty outside."

I freeze for a second, then have to scramble after her to catch up. "Are you serious? Peeing in a horse's stall?"

"Have you ever seen a horse pee? Do you think they care about your little quarter-cup of urine?"

"Wait a minute ... how do you know it's a quarter cup?"

"Oh! My Science Fair topic was about factors influencing urinary output."

"Of course it was ..."

"Uh-huh. I made it to Regionals."

"Of course you did ..."

She throws me a sideways look. "What do you mean by that?"

"I just mean you're a very interesting person, Sasha."

"Well, thanks! Here we are. If you like I'll stay outside while you de-hay yourself."

***

I don't undress completely.

I just undo my breeches and peel them down, inside-out, around my knees so I can give them a really good shake. A small hay / dust cloud forms around the bottom part of my body.

It's as I'm pinging the elastic of my underwear in an attempt to flick out all organic debris that I clue in to Lucas. He's standing, staring, head tilted sideways, ears cupped forward.

"I know, I know." I straighten, tug my cotton bikinis back in place, and reach for the waistband of my breeches. "This is weird for you – I get it. If it's any consolation, it's weird for me, too."

I swear his head nods.

"And also, just for the record, you are *not* the first guy I thought I'd have watching me undress."

A giggle floats through the air.

"Sasha! You're supposed to be giving me privacy!"

She jumps around the corner. "I said I wouldn't look. I never said I wouldn't *listen*."

"Well, there you are now, looking!"

"Pff … I'm looking at you snapping up your breeches. Big whoop."

"Big whoop? Who says that?"

"I do. In fact, when I have my first full-sized horse, his show name is going to be 'Big Whoop.' Whaddya think?"

I think she makes me smile. But I'm not going to tell her that. "I think we should get moving."

"Hey, I'm not the one standing around in my underwear."

***

We go on a hack.

It throws me for a loop when Laney first suggests it. "Bella's mom just texted me to say she's sick, and Terence's family is away this week, so it's just you two," she says, pointing to the remaining small girl on her small pony, and me. "I think we should go on a hack."

I'm puzzled, nervous, and uncertain. First I was told to learn "posting," and, yeah, now that I know what it is, I guess I can see why it's called that. I've been told one day I'll have to learn "cantering." I mean, every human being knows what it means to gallop a horse, but who ever knew there was this weird, in-between gait which I've now learned is something most riders do in most rides, with galloping a comparatively rare activity.

"Hacking" has me stumped. Any definition that comes to mind has no horse connections whatsoever, but the suggestion makes Sasha mutter, "Yes!" under her breath, and sends her into a little flurry of clapping, so it must be OK.

Laney's looking at me with one eyebrow up so I say, "Um, sure. Fine."

"OK," she says. "Sasha, you can get Oreo ready so you can pony Avery." Don't even ask me what ponying is – Sasha's the one who has to do it, so I'm not about to try to figure it out. "As for you Ellie, Lucas is rock-solid so you can just stay behind me, and you'll be fine."

It's reassuring to know I'll be fine. I just wish I knew what I'll be fine doing.

***

It's a trail ride. I mean, that's what I'd call it anyway.

We leave the stable yard and follow a well-worn path around the paddocks. Occasionally the horses behind the fences lift their heads to watch us go by, and at one point all the horses participate in an equine call-and-response session, trading whinnies. Lucas lets out a ringing neigh and I'm amazed how it takes most of his body to produce the sound – it doesn't just come from his head as I expected, but his ribcage expands, and back lifts – the sound vibrates through me as it leaves his body.

For a few brief moments we walk along a ditch beside the road. A car slows as it passes us and Laney lifts a hand to the driver. "She's thinking, 'I wish that was me,'" Laney says.

The thought puffs my chest and lifts my shoulders. It *is* me. I'm riding a horse in the countryside. It's a special thing, and something I couldn't imagine doing just weeks ago.

The trail enters a wooded area. The trees change everything – they block the sun so the temperature drops by noticeable degrees, and amplify the sounds of the birds and of our horses' hooves rustling the thick layer of built-up pine needles topped with more recent fallen leaves.

As we round a corner Laney twists in her saddle. "There's a really low branch ahead. Lean low against Lucas's neck and you'll be fine."

It's a funny thing that as soon as I put my head level with Lucas's neck, I want to hug him. My arms go around him automatically. He strides ahead good-naturedly, even with me – a human limpet – clinging in a most off-balance way. With the branch far behind us I straighten and scratch his withers. "Good boy."

We do lots of new things. Walk up, then down, a small hill. Splash through puddles. Confront a deer.

Being out here with the horses is so completely different from anything I've ever done in my life that it's impossible for any other part of my life to intrude. Just a wide-open field in front of me, and a good horse under me.

"OK?" Laney asks.

"Perfect," I say.

***

We ride back into the stable yard and Avery's mother steps forward. "Well, don't you all look happy!"

Happy, yes. Also, as I discover when I dismount, muddy.

I guess there are consequences to splashing through puddles.

I guess I'll take them.

Sasha catches me looking at Lucas's mud-spattered legs. "Ah, don't worry about that. Groom the rest of him first to let the mud dry, then it'll just flick off."

Sasha is lovely. She's sweet and patient. I'm pretty sure I wasn't as kind as her when I was twelve, and I definitely wasn't as smart.

I'd like to do something nice for her, and I think I know what she'd like.

It's a bonus that it might also keep my big sister on the right side of sanity.

"I'll groom Oreo in his stall, and you can take the cross-ties," Sasha offers. I don't even try to argue with her – I've become good at grooming Lucas when he's immobilized, but I have a mental image of me chasing him around his stall with a hoofpick in my hand. Not dignified.

It's yet another example of Sasha's super-human, un-tweenlike niceness.

"Um, Sasha?"

Her head pops up over the half-door of Oreo's stall. "Yup?"

"You know you said you've never been to a wedding?"

"That's right."

"Would you like to go to one?"

"Huh?!?"

"My sister's wedding. She needs a lead flower girl, and there's even a dress that comes with the job, and it's yours if you want it."

"*What?* Are you seriously *serious?*"

"I wouldn't joke about it."

"Wow! Wow ... I'm suddenly even excited about wearing a dress."

"The only thing is, it's soon. We'll have to see if the dress needs to be altered for you and, if so, we'll have to get it done quickly."

"Oh my gosh!" she says. "Ohmygosh-ohmygosh-ohmygosh. I can't wait to tell my mom. I can't wait to go to a real, actual wedding."

"So that's a yes?"

"As long as my mom says it's OK." Oreo shoves his nose over her shoulder and she tickles his muzzle. "Hey, cookie-boy, I'm going to a *wedding!*"

"There's only one thing," I say.

"What is it?"

"No talking about urine science fair projects."

Sasha winks. "As if I would!"

I lift one eyebrow.

"OK, well, I won't. Promise." She reaches her hand into the aisle. "Pinky swear."

I hook my pinky through hers, then bend down by Lucas's legs. So there it is: I'm bringing someone to Melinda's wedding. And, while I acknowledge it's not exactly what Rachel had in mind, maybe it's good enough to let me keep one of my new paddock boots.

Chapter Fourteen

"You look pretty!" Of course Paige is my nicest sister, but then Rachel backs her up. "You do ... by some complete miracle, because these really are godawful dresses."

Melinda whirls around – or tries to – but lucky for Rachel she's quite literally pinned in place by the seamstress. "Watch it ..." she growls instead.

Rachel has hip-checked me out of the viewing area of the mirror. "I had no idea these straps would look so terrible." She fingers the thick bands of fabric coming over each of her thin, athletic shoulders. "I mean, maybe if I had some double-Ds that needed to be held up ..." She cups her definitely not double-Ds to demonstrate how little support her chest requires. "Hey, I don't suppose you want to trade dresses?" she asks me.

Nobody ever said my sister doesn't have nerve.

I laugh. "No way am I giving up my long sleeves now. Did you see the frost this week?" When my sisters elbowed me out for the skimpier styles of the bridesmaid dresses, the sun was still warming the days to twenty degrees plus, and it hadn't dipped below ten overnight.

These days we're lucky to hit double digits during the brightest part of the day.

Rachel turns to Paige, who looks quite nice in her short-sleeves, and I speak up. "No way. Don't even ask her." Paige's boyfriend has invited her to dinner with his parents. While the two of them are in this happy-happy phase of their relationship I want my sister to look and feel as pretty as she can.

"Aarrgghh!" Rachel says. "I didn't think I'd have the worst dress."

"No, you thought I would."

"Why do you care anyway? Does this mean you have someone to impress? Have you finally found a date for the wedding?"

There's no point in engaging with my sister on this topic – she's too quick, and too cutting, and too much for me to handle. Whatever she throws out, I won't have anything to throw back.

I sidestep out of her way, moving in front of the mirror where I can pretend I'm desperate to get a look at my dress and, to my own considerable surprise, my sisters were right; the dress is OK.

I wouldn't even mind having Terrell see me in it.

The mirror catches the pinking of my cheeks and I turn away before my sisters can notice.

***

Because my parents have been invited to a sixtieth birthday party this evening, the rest of us are able to squish into Rachel's small apartment.

Rachel always says it's the size of her place that keeps her from hosting, but there's black lacy underwear on the arm of the sofa, a package of condoms (fortunately unopened) on the windowsill of the bathroom, and her bed looks like it's never once been made.

My sister can't invite my mom here, because she'd spend the first forty-five minutes cleaning; no doubt finding things no mother should ever find in her daughter's home. The three of us are safer. Melinda will complain loudly, but not touch a thing. Paige will genuinely not notice. Bill, when Melinda brings him, is happy with a beer and the TV remote. I, as always, am quiet. Trying not to rock the boat.

Rachel doesn't even order pizza for us – I'm the one who calls the order in. After the delivery guy leaves, the compact living room fills with conversation:

Melinda: "Can you believe Bill's cousin thought she could bring her dog to my wedding?"

Paige: "Well, it *is* a purse dog."

Rachel: "I'd rather sit next to the purse dog than beside old Aunt Enid."

I'm happy to enjoy my dinner and re-run the last few days. Getting another essay back with a good mark:

reassuring. Learning to do rising trot on Lucas: satisfying. Running into Terrell and maybe, kind of, sort of, asking him to do something that might be perceived as a date: exciting, confusing, pulse-racing.

Terrell. Is the run a date? Will he think so? It is appropriate to try to have a first kiss after an outing that involves mutual sweating?

"Ellie?"

Whoops. Everybody's staring at me.

Huh? What? "Yes?"

"Well, are you?" The intensity of Melinda's stare stirs the devil in me.

I open my eyes wide. "Am I bringing a purse dog to your wedding?"

"Oh, God, Ellie. I'm glad it's a joke to you. Seriously, now that you're bringing your little friend to the wedding, I'm assuming you don't need another seat as well."

It's interesting how quickly me finding a replacement flower girl to save her ceremony, turned into me bringing a friend to the wedding.

I'm not going to answer her. It wasn't even phrased as a question. I lift a slice of pizza to my lips and she cuts in, "Put. The. Pizza. Down. You can eat after you answer me."

It pisses me off. Not only did I order the pizza – I paid for it too and she's had at least two more slices than me. She chose ugly bridesmaid dresses for us while selecting a gown for herself – vintage Fortuny silk – which even my sporty self adores. Just this week I found out there isn't one, single vegetarian option on the wedding menu.

And now she wants to take away my plus-one?

I don't think so. "I'm bringing someone."

The room goes quiet. Melinda is the first to recover. "Excuse me?"

I put my fork down. "Why is this astonishing? Everybody else is bringing somebody."

I know this for a fact, because while we were waiting for the pizza Rachel told us she's invited a guy she met while at a paintball team-building event. "How do you even know what he looks like?" Paige asked. "Doesn't everybody wear masks?"

Rachel sighed. "No he *works* there, dummy."

"Nice prospects then ..." Melinda chimed in.

Rachel put her hand on her hip. "Should we talk about your fiancé? About how he only has his fantastic job because his dad owns the firm?"

That's how I'd ended up paying for the pizza. I'd removed myself from the debate by answering the doorbell, while thinking, *Great. At the wedding everyone else will be with someone so I'll have to play peacemaker.*

Definitely not. I'm going to bring my own guest.

"Who? The Invisible Man? Your imaginary friend from when you were five? He was cute ..." Rachel makes a point of dropping her gaze from my eyes to my feet. Even though I'm not wearing the riding boots, we both know exactly what she means.

"Rachel!" Paige whacks Rachel with her paper plate.

I fold my arms. "You know what? I don't like the tone of this discussion. You don't need to know who I'm bringing." I turn to Melinda. "Just know I *am* bringing somebody so you *can't* have the seat."

Melinda straightens and her eyebrows lift. "I'm sorry, but *whose* wedding is this, Miss-High-and-Mighty?" I'm pretty sure she's not done, but in the absence of our mother, Paige assumes the maternal role.

"Well, I know who's paying for the dinner, Melinda, and I'm pretty sure if you want the charges to stay on Mom's credit card, she's going to say each one of us can bring a guest."

Melinda and Rachel may make the most noise, but when Paige sees fit to chime in, it's best not to mess with her.

Melinda gives me a *This isn't over* look but changes tack, "Well, Paige, speaking of guests, and commitments, Bill's been wondering if your new boyfriend will be joining their bachelor outing. Right Bill?"

The look on Bill's face tells me he's just as unprepared as I was earlier to be pulled into this conversation. But, mouth full of pizza, he takes the easy way out, and nods, and mumbles, "Mm-hm, right."

Meanwhile I leave the room with the excuse of going to the kitchen to wash my hands, trying to retain the satisfaction of having won the plus-one contest with Melinda.

***

Rachel drives me home. She's just pulled into the driveway when our phones give loud bings at exactly the same time.

"Oh God," she says. "Melinda doesn't waste any time, does she?"

She pulls her phone out of the side door pocket of the car and says, "As threatened, the three options for our pre-wedding sisters' brunch. Keep in mind we're going to end up picking up the tab for this, so let me see …"

She's scrolling, clicking, sighing, tutting.

Meanwhile I'm staring at a message which is not from my big sister.

Terrell: **Just got word from Coach. I have practice in the afternoon, but anytime in the morning works. We on?**

I'm amazed Rachel can't hear my heart thumping as I contemplate seeing Terrell twelve hours from now.

She's clueless, though. "OK, I've had a quick look at all the menus. Pick Abacus."

"Huh?"

"I know, I know – why would you even name a restaurant Abacus? So pretentious. But I've been to The Juniper Exchange, and you literally cannot hear yourself think in there, and the other one – Podium – is ..." She rubs her fingers and thumbs together, "... très, très cher."

Her words are bouncing off me, but saying, "OK," seems reasonable.

"Ellie!"

"Yes?"

"Abacus. I said choose that one."

"I ... OK." I look back at my phone and text, **Tomorrow morning is fine.**

"Ellie! What's wrong with you? Did you hear me?"

"No, what did you say?"

"I said, pick the 9:30 a.m. sitting. It won't be as busy. And they increase the price of all the dishes after 11:00."

I add, **9:30 is good for me.**

"Quick!" Rachel's saying. "Send it! That way, even if Paige chooses wrong, you and I will have our picks in first."

I send it.

So. That's done.

Rachel lifts her hand to the ignition, then lets it fall away again, instead using her index finger to poke my arm. "FYI, twelve-year-old flower girls do not count – are we clear?"

My phone vibrates and I glance down to read, **Send me your address and I'll see you at 9:30 tomorrow.**

I lift my eyes to Rachel. "Crystal."

"Are you smiling?"

"Nope. Not smiling. Not me. Quaking in my paddock boots."

She narrows her eyes. "There's something different about you. I'm starting to think you might surprise me."

"I guess we'll see," I say.

"I guess we will." Rachel beeps a quick good-bye as she backs onto the street and I remember I'd better text Melinda **I vote Abacus at 9:30.** before I get in big, big trouble with my sister.

Chapter Fifteen

Sunday morning the chirping of a bird wakes me up. I've had tonnes of sleep, but not too much.

An hour until Terrell gets here.

When I go downstairs for breakfast I find cherries in the fruit bowl. Cherries. At this time of year. It's as decadent as having chocolate truffles for breakfast, but much, much healthier.

I feel great. Can't wait to run.

I have a new pair of running leggings – still with the tags on – that I bought at an end-of-winter sale back in the spring and when I snip the tags off, and pull them on, they fit even better than I remembered.

Perfect.

I brush my teeth ... *minty fresh* ... wash my face, smooth on the super-strength sunscreen all Acnegon users have to apply ... *love this stuff – it's so smooth* ... then contemplate, pony tail or braid?

Let's see ... I lift a comb to my hairline to see how a French braid started just there would look, and, "Ow!"

No way.

I drop the comb in the sink.

Please, please, no.

Lean right in, part the hair – more gently this time, using my fingers – and, sure enough. A big, painful lump is swelling just covered by my hairline.

All the air whistles out of me. Panic replaces it.

No, no, no. I can't. My skin *just* cleared up. Just.

This is my fault. I was too cocky. I started thinking I "used to" have bad skin. I felt sorry for Addy.

And now … it's all going to come back.

I poke at the bump and it really hurts. That's going to be my whole face soon.

Again.

And – oh God – Terrell's going to be here any minute.

I can't go running with him. There's no point. I can't start something with him now. It would be like I'm tricking him. He'd think I'm one way and then I'd turn out to be totally different, and I'd get dumped again …

How do I get rid of him, though?

"Shit!"

"Nice language." I whirl around to face Rachel.

"What are you doing here?"

She puts her finger in front of her lips. "Don't tell Mom, but she and Dad told me they were going out to the garden centre early this morning, and I'm supposed to be hosting a margarita party this afternoon, so I came over to borrow her blender."

"Rachel, that blender's only six months old. She had to buy it after you broke her last one ..." I stop. My mom's blender is the least of my concerns.

"In my defence, the last blender ..."

I smack the counter. "Shut up!"

"What?"

"I couldn't care less about the blender."

"Ellie? What's going on?"

I pull back my hair, point to the bump which I keep hoping will be gone, but seems bigger each time it's exposed to oxygen. I'm angry, panicked, worked up, but all I can manage is a whisper. "It's coming back."

Then the doorbell rings.

I grab Rachel's shoulders. "You have to answer that. You have to get rid of him. Say I'm sick in bed or something. You're good at lying ... you'll come up with something good."

"Do you really think I'm good at lying?"

"Go!" I shove her toward the stairs.

She's back in two minutes.

"Is he gone?"

She stares at me. I've rarely seen my sister look shell-shocked. It's quite alarming.

"What? What is it? What did you tell him?"

"That's Terrell Campbell."

"Yes, I know it is. Which is why ..." I point at what's starting to feel like a horn on my head.

"Ellie. Terrell Campbell is waiting for you downstairs. I don't think you understand what this means. He averages ten points per game. He looks way better close up than he does on the basketball court. He's really polite. And, apparently, he's here to go running with you. Do you know how many people *wish* he would show up on their front doorstep on a Sunday morning?"

"Rachel. Not. Making. Me. Feel. Better."

"Here." It's her turn to take my shoulders. She guides me to the toilet. "Sit down."

"I ..." Whatever. You can't protest Rachel. I sit. "What did you tell him?"

She whips something out of her back pocket, hands it to me. "Pull this over your head."

"It's Mom's tennis visor."

"I know – I grabbed it from the front hall."

"I don't wear visors."

"You do today." She yanks the visor down so it's around my neck and starts brushing my hair using none-too-gentle strokes.

"Ow! You are *not* good at this!"

She tsks. "Mom was too soft with you because you were the baby. I have permanent marks on my scalp from when she used to put my hair in ponytails." Rachel's roughness continues as she twists an elastic into my hair and yanks hard to pull the whole thing tight.

"Look at me," she says.

I do, while asking again, "What did you ..."

"I said you'd be a few minutes. I told him you just painted your toenails and you couldn't put your socks on until they dried."

"Why on earth did you tell him that?"

"Sorry, did you want me to tell him you're freaking out about absolutely nothing – literally one, tiny pimple which is probably from one, single, solitary in-grown hair, that isn't going to multiply, or spread, and does not signify the return of acne at all?" She drops down in front of me and looks me in the eye. "Because that is what this is, Ellie. I promise. It's fine."

I blink. Sniff. Fight hard to breathe. "Oh, Rach. It's so scary."

She pulls me tight to her. "I know it is baby sister. But trust me. The worst part about watching you have acne was watching you not having a life. Terrell Campbell is down there waiting for you. Please, please live your life."

I mumble into her shoulder. "You must love me to confront your toilet-germ-phobia enough to hug me like this."

She mumbles back. "There are times in life when we all have to do things that terrify us."

She backs away and pulls me to my feet. Places me in front of the mirror and adjusts the visor so it hugs my hairline and frames my face. The high pony tail swinging out from behind it looks jaunty and perky. "So?"

"So, OK, I admit it looks cute. But, having a sweaty visor against it isn't exactly going to help my zit go away."

Rachel rolls her eyes. "Are you familiar with the phrase 'short-term pain for long-term gain?' Or, wait, maybe 'you gotta do what you gotta do,' would be more apt. Whatever it is, you run your little heart out, and as soon as you get home you take it off, and wash your hair, and it will all be good ... oh, and maybe try to wash the visor before Mom figures out you borrowed it without asking, and sweated all over it?"

"Well, you would be the Queen of knowing about borrowing things without asking."

Rachel snaps her fingers. "The blender! Thanks for reminding me!"

***

I go downstairs to face Terrell prepared to fake it. Just wanting to get through the run so I can come home and get in the shower.

But it's great.

The temperature is perfect. "Aren't these the days you dream of when you're trying to run in thirty-five-degree humidity in July?" Terrell asks.

"Yes! I'm so happy you think that, because everyone else is all, 'Oh, it's getting colder. Oh, I wish summer was back,' but I love this time of year."

"Fall is my favourite season," he says.

"Me, too."

Then, as we power along my favourite path running behind Parliament, with the legendary river on one side and the sheer cliffs on the other, he says, "Really, does it get any better than this?"

"I know," I say. "I feel lucky every time I get to do this run."

"Yeah. Most people think I stayed here for the basketball program – which, I mean, is great – but really, this is my home. I love this place."

I smile and he says, "What?"

"Nothing, really. Just I'm really glad I came on this run."

He laughs. "I am, too. There was a moment there, with the toenail polish, when I wondered, but – *phew!* – it all turned out fine."

***

By the time we stop running I've already found out that Terrell also has three older sisters.

"But have you been through the hell that is wedding planning?" I ask.

He wags a finger at me. "Wedding planning is for wusses. Wait until you witness the hoopla around the production of the first grand-child."

He knows I used to play ringette, and have just started horseback riding.

"I've always wanted to ride a horse," he says.

"You know, my mom said the same thing. Even though my best friend is a rider, I'd never considered it, but now I'm hooked."

It's not overwhelming when he says, "Maybe you could take me riding someday?" because the day when I would ever be competent enough to take somebody else riding is so far in the distant future that it's easy to say, "Maybe."

"Just not next week, because I'm leaving town."

"Where are you going?"

He makes a face. "The classic 401 tour of Southern Ontario. A bunch of pre-season games."

I've played my fair share of ringette games in the area around Toronto – if you play sports in Ontario it's a trip you're going to make at some time. I recall the traffic jams and the heaving roadside service centres. I remember hotel parking lots with no empty spaces. "I know what you mean ... although, I might trade with you just this once."

"Oh yeah? Why?"

"That wedding I mentioned. It's coming up – and there will be last-minute wedding madness until it happens. You should see the dress I have to wear."

"I think I'd like to see that dress." And, just like that, we're not just casually chatting. There's something in Terrell's tone that sets off butterflies in my stomach. There's something in it that makes me drop our eye contact.

I should, look at him though. This is my moment to say, "There's something I'd like to ask you." I haven't been Rachel's little sister all these years without figuring out this guy has just given me an opening. If I was ever going to invite him to Melinda's wedding, this would be the time.

With the casual easiness of our conversation interrupted, I have time to think. To doubt and second-guess. My finger wanders to the edge of the visor right where it's covering my burgeoning pimple. Who knows what I'll look like by the day of the wedding? Who knows what I'll look like for the foreseeable future?

I force myself to laugh. "Well, my sister all but admitted she chose terrible dresses for us so she'd look better by comparison, so you probably don't want to see it."

"Hmm … yeah. I've heard of people doing that." He seems fine. Still friendly. Still smiling.

It's not that I don't like him. I really, really do. I just got a bit shaken this morning. I just need to watch my skin over the next few days. I have an appointment with Dr. Hamilton coming up – it's supposed to be one of my last ones – after I talk to her maybe I'll feel better, braver.

There's nothing saying I can't still ask Terrell to the wedding.

I just can't do it this morning.

Chapter Sixteen

By the time Sunday dinner with my sisters rolls around, I'm feeling pretty Zen. I always feel best after physical exertion and my run with Terrell was long and satisfying. I got a surprising amount of homework done. The pimple is still there, but no bigger, and Rachel's explanation that it's an in-grown hair seems plausible.

Terrell and I really hit it off. Our conversation was great. And, yeah, I admit it, I didn't have the guts to ask him out, but next time … maybe next time.

So, I can handle family dinner.

Until Melinda takes us deep into the wedding weeds.

Each week the amount of time we're able to eat before wedding talk begins decreases in inverse relation to the amount of time left before the wedding.

Tonight I've had two forkfuls of salad, and one of lasagna, before the details start rolling. Melinda's university roommate and her husband have canceled, now, when it's too late to get a refund on their two already-purchased dinners.

"Wow!" Rachel says. "Did she at least give a reason?"

"Oh, something about preeclampsia and her obstetrician wanting her on bed rest ..."

"That's actually pretty serious," Paige says.

"Yeah? Well so is my wedding."

Through a stroke of good fortune, Melinda did a drop-in visit on the venue and discovered they were planning to use the wrong shade of tablecloths. She shakes her head. "Wheat, instead of flax. Can you believe it? You can't trust anyone to do a good job."

I try to just eat quietly and nod in the right places. I'm afraid if I do anything to draw attention to myself, I'll end up being the one sent to the wedding planning place to bring back samples of the new tablecloths and then deliver them to the venue which is actually farther away than Laney's barn.

"It's exclusive," Melinda had said when we'd raised the driving time needed to get there.

"It's remote," Rachel had said.

It's Melinda's wedding, so Melinda gets what she wants, but the rest of us do our best not to be sent on errands that involve driving the forty-five-minute drive to the venue.

When my mom dishes up the last serving of lasagna, I see my chance. I reach for the now-empty casserole dish. "Let me take that. It needs to be soaked."

To my surprise, as soon as I'm up, I'm not the only one holding the dish. Rachel, who came in a taxi with a glow about her I'm assuming was generated by at least a couple of afternoon margaritas, has a firm grip on it as well. "I'll help too!"

I give it a tug, but she's holding tight. "What are you doing?" I hiss.

She flicks her chin toward the kitchen and returns my hiss. "Get in there."

As soon as we're around the corner she lifts her hands away from the dirty dish. "Now that is going to take some elbow-grease." She leans against the counter. "I'd recommend you get started."

"Rachel, what's going on? Did you break the blender? Because I'm not going to cover for you ..."

"How was your run?"

I focus my attention on the lasagna dish since I have no margaritas to explain away my warm cheeks. "It was good."

"*Good* ... come on, Ellie!"

While I'm buying time by squirting detergent in the bottom of the dish, Rachel suddenly gasps. "Oh my God! That basketball game you went to with Lucas ... *that* was when you met Terrell Campbell, wasn't it?"

I turn the hot water on full and turn to my sister. "Lucas knows him from club ball. He introduced us after that game. We both run, so ..." I shrug. "No big deal."

"*We both run.* What's that supposed to mean? Every human being runs, but not everybody runs together on a Sunday morning. I can't believe what perfect timing this is – you met him just in time to bring him to Melinda's wedding."

"That's a bit premature."

"How old are you Ellie? 'Premature?' Geez, girl. Act your age. Jump that boy's bones. Be the person with the best-looking date at the wedding. Upstage the bride."

"All in that order?"

"Ellie ... Why wouldn't you? He's gorgeous. *Gorgeous.* Did I mention gorgeous? And such a good ball player. And, we had the team in for a profile we did for the alumni magazine last year and he was so nice. And he organized that fundraiser last year – what was it called? – 'Hoop there it is' and the proceeds went to subsidize club basketball for kids who wouldn't be able to afford it otherwise ..."

I reach out and slam off the faucet. "I get it Rach. He's perfect. Noted. Which is exactly why it was just a run." I turn away from my sister and begin organizing dirty dishes like my life depends on it. *This can soak in the casserole dish. This can go in the dishwasher.*

Arms circle my waist. Slender, but surprisingly strong. Like twin bands of steel. Then my sister's chin digs into my shoulder. "Ellie. I wasn't telling you those things so you'd think he was too good for you. I was letting you know I actually think he's good enough."

I stand still for a minute while I let her words sink in. I turn, still in her arms, and put my own arms around her and give her a squeeze "That's a surprisingly nice thing for you to say."

She pulls me even tighter and says, "You have to promise to tell me if he's a good kisser!"

It's good to know some things never change.

***

Dinner over. Dishes washed. Sisters gone. The house is quiet. I'm finishing the Legal Studies assignment I started with Addy when my laptop notifies me I have messages.

Fittingly the first one is from Addy. **I think I'm done my part of the assignment. I'm attaching it here for you to look over. Let me know what you think.**

Then there's a message from Dr. Hamilton's office. An automated reminder of my upcoming appointment. **Click to confirm** it requests. I triple-click.

And now it's time for me to finish my part of the assignment and send it over to Addy. I reading it over, trying to get my head back into rhythm of Legal Studies, when my phone pings.

It'll be Melinda asking me to pick up tablecloth swatch samples after all. Or Rachel telling me Paige chose the wrong brunch restaurant and now we're all doomed to go to some place called "Swank" or "Posh" where orange juice costs sixteen dollars and all the omelettes are made with quail eggs.

My phone has assigned all my sisters pink contact icons, which irritates Rachel – "Why don't you change mine?" she asked. "Can you think of anyone less pink than me?" – but figuring out how to change it seems like too much of an effort, and I'm used to them as pink, so I leave it. The icon attached to this new text is not pink – it's quite a nice shade of blue. I don't think any of my other contacts are this exact colour.

Great run. Thank you.

It's Terrell.

Oh. Wow. That makes me feel good.

Maybe Rachel is right. Or at least partly right.

I need to find a way to ask that boy to the wedding.

Bonus if I can do it in a way that I won't have to face Rachel's gloating.

Chapter Seventeen

I figured it would be a one-off when Rachel took me to my first appointment with Dr. Hamilton.

I completely appreciated her doing it – truth is I wouldn't have gone without her, and I was really happy she sat in and listened to all the information because it was all so overwhelming to me I couldn't remember most of it on my own.

But with appointments once a month for the better part of a year, and Rachel's work so busy, and her not exactly being the nurturing type, I knew I could ask my mom to drive me or, for that matter, I could bus it. I mean, if Dr. Hamilton drove four hours for her dermatologist appointments when she was a teenager, I could use public transit, even if it did require making a couple of transfers.

I was really surprised when Rachel went to the window on our way out of the office after the first appointment and asked, "Could you make our next appointment also on a Wednesday around noon? This time works really well for me to bring my sister."

The last Wednesday of every month ever since Rachel and I have driven out to Dr. Hamilton's office. We figured out we can avoid the parking fees in medical building's parking lot by leaving the car next door in one of the spaces of the Lebanese grocery store that also sells amazing Mediterranean pies. When I asked Rachel "Is it really fair to park here?" she said, "Of course – where do you think we're going to buy our lunch afterwards?"

So we have a routine of a dermatology appointment, followed by a Mediterranean pie, and I've come to quite like it. As we climb the three storeys to Dr. Hamilton's office I'm thinking I'll miss this when I stop coming but it will be good for Rachel to be able to reclaim her Wednesdays at lunch.

As usual we're called in for our appointment right on time, and as usual, Rachel nods in satisfaction.

I sit on the examination table; an awkward teenager wearing ripped jeans with paper crinkling under my backside every time I move, and Rachel settles into the chair in the corner, hanging her smooth leather tote from the arm.

She takes her phone, turns it off, slips it in her bag, and looks up at me.

"You always do that," I say.

"Do what?"

"Turn your phone off when we're here."

"Ellie," she says. "This is one of the most relaxing moments in my month. Nobody knows where I am, nobody can call me, I can't get any messages, and, if anyone does try to reach me I have the best excuse in the world for not being available."

"Oh." I'd never thought of it that way. That my go-getter sister might need an escape every now and then. Certainly never thought coming here with me would provide it. "What are you going to do when my appointments are done?"

She smiles. "We're going to pretend they're not. Last Wednesday of every month. You and me, kid. It's staying in my calendar. Start coming up with ideas."

I'm laughing when Dr. Hamilton pushes the door open and she stops dead and stares at me. "Oh my goodness, Ellie Hannaman. Aren't you a picture?"

Dr. Hamilton tells us she's pleased, but not surprised, by my progress. "Everyone sees results at different times, and you did have to be a bit patient, but look at you, Ellie – wasn't it worth it?"

I tell her about my "slight anxiety" over the pimple in my hairline. Rachel helpfully chimes in, "Um, it was more like a complete meltdown."

"You're doing fine." Dr. Hamilton tells me. "You'll continue to do fine. Anxiety is normal. I wish I could give you something to take that all away for you, but that's something you'll have to work on for yourself. It's hard, but you can do it."

She types up my next prescription. "If all goes well at your next appointment, this will be your final prescription," and when she stands up her foot hits my right paddock boot which has tipped over onto the floor. "Hardcore boots," she says.

"Aren't they?" Rachel asks. "I bought them for her when she started horseback riding."

"Really?" Dr. Hamilton asks.

"Well, yeah," Rachel says. "She was using my hundred-and-fifty-dollar designer rubber boots. I had to get them back."

"Those boots cost a hundred and fifty dollars?" I ask Rachel. "They were more than the paddock boots!"

"Ladies!" Dr. Hamilton holds her hand up. "I'm not actually that interested in the boots." She turns to me. "You started horseback riding?"

I nod. "Right after Labour Day."

"Well, now that is interesting. I think that's something a lot of people dream of trying, but never quite know how to start. Would you consider letting me showcase you in one of my newsletters?"

"One of your newsletters?"

"I'm not sure if you read them, but I like to have interesting stories about patients who've completed their treatment with me, and what they're doing. We usually have stories lined up several months in advance, so the timing would work well – you'd be done your treatment and we could showcase your adventures in horseback riding."

"But ... but ..."

"You don't have to decide right this minute." She scribbles a phone number on a card and hands it to me. "This is my cell number. Text me and remind me to send you the list of questions we use. Once you see them you can decide if you'd want to be featured."

"But the people in your newsletters have all done amazing things."

Rachel leans forward. "Ellie. Dr. Hamilton is trying to tell you that you're amazing. Say thank you."

"I ... um ... thank you."

The doctor smiles. "My pleasure. I hope you'll decide to participate. Text me. And I'll see you both next month."

As Rachel and I cross the parking lot to the Lebanese bakery I say, "Can you believe she wants to write about me in one of her newsletters?"

Rachel sighs. "Of course I can, Ellie. Just like I also knew that little pimple was no big deal." She hip checks me. "Seriously, Ellie, you owe me big-time. I give you great advice but you never believe it until other people tell you."

I open my mouth to protest and instead find myself saying, "You're right, Rach. Let me buy you a meat pie to make up for it."

Chapter Eighteen

Saturday morning. I'm sitting at the bottom of the stairs, pulling on my riding boots, when a shadow falls across the glass pane in the door.

It won't be a door-to-door salesperson because they go to the front door – which is why we don't answer the front door. If it's one of my sisters, she'll walk right in. It's probably our neighbour from across the street who mostly lives in a condo paid for by his company in downtown Toronto. He tends to arrive home late at night, only to wake up in the morning and realize he has no milk.

I suppress a sigh as I stand up to check. If it's him I'll have to take off the boot I've already laced up so I can go back into the kitchen for the milk.

I peer through the window and yell, "*Em!*"

I whip the door open and she laughs, and I grab her, and we hug and yell things like, "I'm so excited to see you!" and "I missed you so much!" and I'm asking, "What are you doing here?" and she's asking, "Can I come to the barn with you?"

"Of course you can come!" I say. "But I need to leave right now."

Em points at her feet, sporting boots just as dusty and broken-in as mine. "I'm ready. Let's go!"

***

I keep looking sideways at Em. She looks the same, of course; it hasn't been *that* long. But there's also a hint of unfamiliarity about her. It's probably a combination of her hair being an inch longer than the last time I saw her, the shirt she's wearing being one I haven't seen before, and maybe it's me, too.

I've never been the one in the driver's seat taking her to the barn. Things look different from this side of the car. I guess they'll look even more different when I'm the one up on her horse.

Which makes me think ... "Listen, Em. You probably want to ride Lucas. I'm sure Laney can put me on another horse for today."

"Don't be silly. I want to see you ride my horse. It's going to be so cool. Besides, I think he's fit enough for me to climb up for a few minutes after you ride."

"If you're sure ..."

She smiles by way of answer, and I remember this about her. Some people find Em difficult. "Prickly" is one of the most polite descriptions I overheard about her in the halls at our high school. But when Em likes you ... loves you ... when Em has your back, there is no better friend in the world.

***

"Wow, you're in – what? – Week Five of riding and you already muck out a stall better than me ..." Em shakes her head. "Impressive."

I'm blushing. I can't believe my cheeks are hot because Em says I have a talent for shoveling manure. But, there you go, I'm undeniably, ridiculously, pleased.

There is something special about Em's approval, though. She doesn't give it easily, so when it comes, it means a lot. As I walk Lucas around the track, I hear her telling Sasha, "You must be a great teacher – look how she's keeping her heels down all the time. None of those kids are doing that." I sneak a glance over my shoulder and see Sasha's face lit up with the praise.

It's nerve-wracking, but rewarding, to ride Em's horse in front of her. Sasha talks me through my paces while Laney works with the younger kids. Today's their first day not being led by their mothers. The one on the smallest, most maniacal pony zips through the middle of my circle at one point, but other than that they keep to their end of the ring.

We're all improving.

When Em's seen everything I've got she claps. "Very, very good!" Lucas's ears prick forward at the sound of her voice and, as he's been doing ever since we got out here, he tries to veer toward her.

This time I let him.

One ear flicks back to me as though he's asking, "Are you really going to let me do this?" then he gives up and breaks into a walk-jog, hustling straight up to Em and thrusting his head against her chest.

She smooths his forelock and pushes her face against the big white marking on his face, and they stay like that as the seconds tick away. When she finally lifts away, I catch the quickest glint of tears in her eyes – so faint, and gone so fast, I might have imagined them. It reminds me that things are sometimes hard for everybody – even the people who seem super-strong.

So remember that next time you think you're the only person with problems.

I figure it's time for Em to mount up, but she wrinkles her nose and says, "OK, so I've seen what you can do, now what are you going to learn today?"

"Oh, I'm good. It was a good review session. You can ride him now."

Em shakes her head. "Nuh-uh. You're halfway through – is that right?" She turns to Sasha, who nods. "No time to rest on your laurels. I'm thinking sitting trot."

Sasha giggles and instead of filling me with joy, apprehension creeps in. It takes a step toward dread when Sasha says, "You thought *rising* trot was hard ..."

"Great ..." I say.

"Hush, both of you," Em says. "You'll do fine, Ellie. Just take him out on the track and get a nice forward walk going."

Em's arms are folded, which means there's no point in saying no. Besides, I know how to walk. I'm a walking expert. Lucas and I walk.

"Now, you're going to ask him to trot, just the way you've been doing, but instead of letting his motion push you into a post, you're going to keep your butt in the saddle and absorb it."

Oh yeah. That sounds easy. Absorb a force strong enough to thrust me out of the saddle. No problem.

"Sorry, I didn't hear you!" Em calls.

"No problem!" I call back.

"I was pretty sure you said that – I just didn't hear it."

Ever since I figured out posting I've had no problem getting Lucas to trot. Since we both know there won't be any teeth-gritting full-on flopping we're happy to do it.

This time is different. The trot ask I make is a mere technicality. I don't put any heart into it. I don't want to go back to being a messy, bouncy trotter, which means I don't really want to trot. Lucas knows it; his ears swing back and he swishes his tail but he doesn't trot.

"Um … what happened there?" Em asks.

"Nothing," I mutter.

"Exactly," she says. "This time make something happen instead."

I ... oh ... I don't want to ...

"Breathe!" Sasha's high, clear voice rings out and I remember how the breathing plan got me over the hump of rising trot, and for six or seven seconds confidence flows through my veins, and that's all it takes for Lucas to obey my ask and move up to the trot.

I immediately start posting.

"*Sitting*, I said!" Em calls.

"You can do it," Sasha adds. "You can keep posting in your head; just not with your hips."

What on earth does she mean?

I rise again.

"Sasha's right!" Em says. "Just decide you're going to stay in the saddle but let your hips move with him."

"And breathe!"

"*Up-down, up-down, up-down ...*" I'm muttering as I pass by the two of them.

"Change it to '*one-two, one-two, one-two ...*'" Sasha advises.

Oh, what the heck. *Next time,* I tell myself. Except I rise again. *OK, this next time.*

One deep breath. *One-two, one-two, one-two* and I'm bouncing. Oh no, I'm all over the place. Oh no, poor Lucas ...

"Absorb!"

"Breathe!"

I exhale, and my pelvis tips forward, then resets.

Then I jiggle for two more strides, before managing one more smooth hip swing.

One rough stride, then two fluid ones.

Concentrate, swing, breathe ... I manage a complete circle with only one rough break and I'm exhausted.

"Walk!" I tell Lucas and he responds instantly. I stroke his neck. "You're a good boy." And that's the absolute truth because he doesn't immediately try to run to Em, he just lets out a long, whiffling exhale and briefly turns his head in my direction and continues walking for me.

Em walks over to meet us. "Great job! Now that you've got the hang of sitting trot you're perfectly set up for canter work."

"Canter?" My eyes find Sasha. "Can't I just enjoy sitting trot for a while?"

She gives me a thumbs up. "Don't worry – you'll be ready and it will be great!"

***

I feel – well, not exactly *great* – but *good* for a few minutes. I mean, this stuff is all new to me. It's not easy but I'm trying anyway. A few minutes watching Laney work with the little kids tells me I'm doing as well as them – maybe better with some things – and learning should be way easier for them. Their bodies are tiny, and flexible, and they have no concept of fear.

So, yeah, maybe I deserve a pat on the back after all.

"Oh, nice ..." Sasha says beside me, and I turn to watch Em, and realize I'm a dog of a rider. I have no idea what I'm doing. I'm actually embarrassed Em saw me ride.

Because, under her, Lucas looks like a different horse. He seriously looks taller. Thinner. Lighter. His feet seem to float and the parts of him that feel solid to me look simply strong with Em on his back.

Muscles show all along his body – from neck to tail – and, even though I'm new to this, I can tell Em's hands, and legs, and heels – those pesky heels it takes all my concentration to keep down – are in exactly the right places.

Em can ride Lucas in tiny, perfectly round circles. She can move him from a half-circle one direction, to a half-circle in the other. She can take him straight from a walk to what I guess is a canter, even though I haven't tried one yet. I can see, though, that there are a lot of things for him to figure out with his body, but Em seems to give him the support and confidence he needs to just go ahead and concentrate on where his legs should go, and they move from the quiet, simple walk to a rocking, energetic pace.

"I will never be able to do that."

Sasha tsks. "Well, duh, as if anyone would ask you to do a walk-canter transition now. It's hard. Oreo and I are still working on ours." She squints as, at the end of the ring Em and Lucas return just as sweetly and calmly to the original walk. "But you will be able to canter and if you stick with it, one day you can do walk-canter."

I shake my head and get a nudge in the ribs. "Yes you will. No doubt."

"As long as I remember to breathe?" I say it lightly, with a joke in my voice.

"Well, it's worked so far, hasn't it?"

And I have to admit – no joke – she has a point.

***

We leave Lucas with minty-fresh breath (Scotch mints are his favourite treat), and a beautifully brushed tail (Em narrowed her eyes at him and predicted, "That won't last long"), ambling down the long path to laze away the rest of his Saturday with the other horses in the herd.

I pull into the gas station. Ever since my mom helped me take these lessons I make sure to take the car back to her with more gas in it than when I left.

Em watches the numbers tick over on the pump and sighs.

"What is it?" I'm watching the pump, too. I only have a ten-dollar bill and I don't want to go over.

"I miss him." She adds, "Lucas," then giggles, "both of them, because now that I'm here, and I've just seen my horse, I miss my boyfriend back at school."

Her words – or maybe the tone behind them – give me a flutter of anxiety. I didn't think it would be on my mind so much, but I keep thinking about Terrell, and especially about him going out of town. I feel like it's created a deadline. Like I can't just let him go without seeing him first. But we didn't make any plans after running, and now I don't know how to. And when I start thinking about it I worry he would have said something if he'd wanted to see me again. But he sent me that nice text ... But that's all he did ...

"Shit!" My concentration's slipped and I stop the pump at $10.37.

Em pokes my side. "What's up Ellie?"

I shrug. "Nothing." I make a big deal of tapping the nozzle off before I hang it up.

"I don't believe you."

"No, really." I'm screwing the gas cap back on.

"Does it have something to do with this?" Em's holding up her phone with the picture of me and Lucas and Terrell at the basketball game.

"Oh!" *Wow, he has a nice smile.* I look at Em, and she says, "Thought so. Let's pick up some lunch on the way home and you can tell me all about it."

I wrinkle my nose. "I literally have no money."

"Lunch is on me."

I wave my single ten-dollar bill under her nose. "Well, you're also going to have to give me thirty-seven cents, otherwise I'll have to stay here and work off my tab.

Chapter Nineteen

"Take me to your school!" Em says.

"What? No. It's not really on the way."

"It's not really out of the way. Plus I hear there's a great food truck there – fish tacos – and I'm buying so I get to decide."

I hesitate. "We can pick up bagels at that place in the village ..."

"... any day of the week," Em finishes. "I want to picture you at school. Come on."

***

We go, and instead of fish tacos, it's the veggie bowl guy parked in the food truck spot, which is my good luck. I take in his dreadlocks, and ear spacers, and the tats encircling his neck like a turtleneck and marvel yet again at Rachel's wide-ranging and eclectic taste in men.

We get our food and Em gives a dramatic shiver. "I can't enjoy eating in single-digit temperatures." She juts her chin toward the Athletic Centre. "Inside."

Although they're different in many ways, Rachel and Em are the same in that you really have to pick your battles with them, because you're going to lose ninety per cent of the time. Even though I'm suspicious of her motives, I'm not going to fight Em on going into the building.

Besides – she's right – it's cold outside.

We have our pick of the tables in the alcove where I worked with Addy, and Sophia, and Olivia, and in the daylight it's lovely, and warm, and sun-filled, and the veggie bowls are delicious, and I smell like horse, and my best friend's with me. It all lulls me into a general state of comfort, complacency, and contentment.

"So," Em says. "Tell me about your love life, and then tell me why you haven't already told me about your love life."

I smush a chick pea between my molars. "How did I know that was coming?"

"Because I love you enough to care, which brings me back to my second question."

OK. I can answer the second question no problem. "*Nobody* knows – well, except Rachel."

"Rachel! You told the least discreet person in the world, and you didn't tell me, and that's supposed to be a consolation?"

"Come on, Em. You know Rachel – do you really think I told her voluntarily?"

"OK, I give you that. Rachel has a way of inserting herself even when not invited. You can make it up to me by making me the first person you tell voluntarily."

"Let me just ... one more bite ..." I fork up noodles, and sesame seeds, and more chick peas in some kind of vegan broth.

"I know, it is amazing, isn't it?" Em's slurping broth from her plastic spoon.

"Rachel slept with him, you know. The veggie bowl guy."

"Oh my God. I wish Rachel was the marrying type. Then he'd be your brother-in-law, and you could have this food all the time." Em swipes a napkin across her mouth. "Enough of that, though. Spill."

I think for a minute. How to tell her? Timeline? Backstory?

Maybe just the basics.

"I think I could really like him – I tap her phone so she'll know we're talking about Terrell – and we had a moment where I could have asked him to Melinda's wedding, and I got in my own way, and I didn't ask, and now ..." I shrug. "Now he's going away in a few days and I probably won't see him before then."

I sometimes forget about the soft side of Em. I expect tough love, Rachel-style. Instead, she leans forward and takes my hand. "Were you afraid to ask because of what happened with Rory?"

I think about that for a minute. It would be easy to blame it on Rory. It would make me the victim. But it probably wouldn't be true – not anymore. Rory's living his life, and I have to live mine. So, I tell the truth. "It was me. I found a zit here –" I dig around in my hairline and have trouble even pinpointing the spot that originally felt like Mount Vesuvius. "– and I went zero-to-sixty. My acne would come back full force, I could never have a social life, the world would end, and so on."

She doesn't say anything for a second, and I say, "Dumb, I know."

"How about 'understandable but unfortunate?'"

"Well, that's definitely nicer than 'dumb.'"

"Also, fixable."

"Pardon me?"

"I said, 'fixable.' As in 'correctable' 'remediable.'" She gathers up her packaging. "Any chance there's a basketball practice on in the gym?"

"Wait, Em ..." Just when I was getting lulled into complacency by the soft, empathetic Em, here's the chop-chop, pitter-patter-let's-get-at-er version of my best friend back in full force.

No surprise, she's not waiting. I shove my food-splattered wrappers into the organic composting bin and run after her.

***

"This is embarrassing." I'm talking to Em's back, since she's two steps ahead of me.

She turns and walks backward, facing me. "Walking through a public building is embarrassing?"

"You know what I mean."

She grins. "You're extra cute when you're embarrassed."

God, she's like Rachel. "Actually I think I might have gotten the date wrong – the team might have already left."

Of course I know that's not true. I have a secret dot on Tuesday on my calendar at home which is the day I know they're leaving. But the lie might be the only way to put Em off.

No such luck. "Then there's obviously nothing to be embarrassed about." Em stops at each set of glass doors and peers in.

"We might as well go."

She shrugs. "Fine. On our way out there's no harm in looking."

"Looking for what?"

Both Em and I whirl around to face Terrell. "Oh! It's you!" I say. "I didn't think you'd be here!"

"Then who were you looking for in the gym?"

I swallow hard. Strive for light, funny, casual. Doing this in front of Em is excruciating. "I wasn't looking for anyone. My poor friend here," I fling my arm out toward Em. "Goes to a substandard university that doesn't have such a nice gym. She's gawking."

Em steps forward. "That's me. I gawk at basketball players." She thrusts her hand out. "I'm Em."

"Lucas's girlfriend," I add.

Terrell laughs. "Ah, so you have your very own basketball player to gawk at."

Em gives a coquettish blink. "Now we just have to make sure Ellie has one too."

I jab her in the side. "Oh, I'm sorry. Did your ribcage just run into my elbow?"

She clutches at her ribs. "My bad. I'll just retreat over here and die quietly, by myself, in the corner."

She returns to her post by the glass doors and gives us a little wave. "I'm sorry," I say. "She likes to stir things up. I tried to back her off by telling her the team had already left, but then you showed up and exposed that lie."

He shakes his head. "Nope, three more sleeps then we're outta here."

"You sound like you can't wait."

Now I swear he's the one fighting down a blush. His cheeks have a suspicious glow to them. "Well ... I mean ... I want to play ... there should be some good games ... but ..."

"But what? It'll be fun."

He shrugs. "I just ..." He takes a deep breath. "It would be cool if you could see a game."

I clap my hand to my breastbone and am about to laugh it off when something in the way he blinks, then looks away, before looking back, makes me realize we're not doing the joking thing anymore. "Well, as much as I'd like to dodge my pre-wedding bridesmaid duties, I don't think I can make it to Southern Ontario. But, next home game?"

"Yeah?"

"I mean, sure, if I can get my hands on a ticket. They're tough to come by."

He grins and the awkwardness is gone. "I think I can find you a ticket. I can probably even get a spare one, too, so you can bring your disadvantaged friend over there ... or anyone you want, of course."

I remember my feeling from before. Of not knowing how to make plans to see him again. And now here he is, standing right in front of me. "That would be great." A little rush of courage prompts me to add, "And maybe after the game we could, I don't know, do whatever you do after you play. Eat? Drink?"

His smile lifts the corners of his eyes and they're such a contrast in dark and white I think I could look at them forever. "I have an even better idea, if you're up for it. Believe it or not, they don't feed us very well on these trips ..."

"Fine-tuned athletic machines like you? I find that hard to believe."

"Sadly, it's true. So I always try to get a really good meal in before I leave. Would you maybe like to come out for dinner with me Monday night?"

Whoa. That's very direct.

It's also completely wipes out my worries about not seeing him before he leaves ...

It also gives me a chance to ask him to the wedding ...

It's also sending butterflies crashing through my stomach ...

Em clears her throat and the only thing worse than me saying the wrong thing would be Em saying it for me.

"I'd like to! I mean, as long as I don't have any huge assignments I'm forgetting about, but it sounds good."

"It does?" he asks.

"It does. Yes. It does. Definitely ... oh, wow, I'm babbling ... sorry ..."

Terrell steps toward me, and slides his right hand under my ear, holding my head steady, then presses his right cheek to mine. He brushes his lips against the skin in front of my ear and whispers, "Don't be sorry."

When he steps back my head is buzzing. "You'd better go now."

"Why?"

"Because Em definitely wants to talk to me about this."

He laughs out loud. "OK, so if my ears are burning, I'll just ignore it." He waves over at Em, and says, "I'll text you on Monday," before leaving.

***

As Em and I step out into the cold, she pulls out the front of her shirt and makes a show of fanning it. "Whoa," she says. "After watching that, I really need to get back to school to see Lucas, if you know what I mean."

I shoot her a look. "Not appropriate."

"Says the girl who basically had sex-with-her-clothes-on in the hallway of the Athletic Centre." She grins and links her arm through mine. "Oh, Ellie. Enjoy it. You deserve it. And am I ever glad we came here for lunch!"

Yeah. Me too.

Chapter Twenty

I step off the bus into the kind of cold, pouring, relentless autumn rain that's the polar opposite of Indian Summer. Instead of reminding me of kinder, gentler times, it sends chill fingers rivuletting under my collar, snaking down my back, telling me, *It's only getting colder from here on in; winter's coming.*

The leaves that crisped under my feet, and swirled away from my flying legs on yesterday's run, form thick boggy layers in the bottom of the puddles that ooze around the soles of my shoes and soak my socks.

Still, as soon as I drop my bag in the front hall and strip off my sopping shoes and socks, I dash upstairs to change into running clothes.

I need to get out.

I need to run fast and hard.

Need to blow out the jitters, clear my head. Figure out little things, like *What should I wear tonight? Do I let him pay? Do I offer?* As well as big things like, *What if he doesn't text me after all? What if he does? What about afterwards?*

By the time I drop to a walk at the corner of my street it's full-on dark. Normally the sun wouldn't be down

quite yet, but with the rain clouds as thick as they are, all the illumination is from streetlights and car headlights. It bounces crazily off the surfaces of puddles and is refracted by the raindrops. It's a night for staying in – for having a long-term boyfriend to cuddle with on the couch and not have to go outside.

But I'll never have a long-term boyfriend if I don't have a first date.

My phone buzzes. **Team meeting just ending. Are we still on? Can I pick you up for dinner?**

Oh. He texted. That's one big question out of the way.

I scoot under the shelter of our front porch roof and with the water sluicing down behind me, tumbling to the walkway like a waterfall, I take out my phone and, in the light of the front porch, text **Yes. Thanks. I'm soaking – just got in from a run in the rain – OK to go after I have a shower?**

As soon as I send it I'm short of breath and I don't know if it makes it worse, or better when I get a near-instant reply. **You can have a shower. You can have two. You can do whatever you like. I'm so happy you're coming. I'll drive home to pack some things, then text you to see if you're ready.**

I guess I'd better hope his packing takes a while because the look I'm currently rocking is drowned rat, and can only be rescued by a long, hot shower followed by a long, hot session with the hair dryer.

Given I might be in the bathroom a while, I bring my phone in with me and decide, other than the phone being here, I'm not going to overthink the dinner thing. Just get cleaned up like it's any old night and enjoy swapping cold and wet for warm and dry.

Drenched running gear literally peeled off me and heaped on the floor, I'm testing the water for my shower when my phone rings.

Unknown number. Local, though. Could Terrell already be home and calling me from his landline? I swipe to answer. "Hello?"

"Oh my God! Ellie! I'm so glad you're there. I didn't know what else to do ... didn't know who to call ..."

"Sasha? Is that you?"

"Yes! It's me. I'm at the barn. O-o-oreo ... Oooo-reo ..."

I crank the roaring water off, and turn her own advice back on her. "Sasha! Breathe!"

"Oh!" She takes a hiccupping breath.

"What's going on, Sasha?"

"Laney called me at home. She had to go into the city this afternoon and she said the traffic's really bad, and there was a pile-up on the highway and she's OK, but the car's damaged and she can't drive it, so she asked me to come over and feed because she doesn't know when she'll get back, and Oreo is ..." Her breathing rate increases again, and becomes audible in short, sharp gasps over the line.

"Oreo's what?"

"I think he's colicking. I'm so scared. I don't know what to do."

Which one hundred per cent makes two of us. In fact, I don't even know what colicking is.

"Sasha, where are your parents?"

"M-m-my dad's in Toronto on business and my mom's gone to choir. They're not allowed to have their cell phones on when they're singing."

Shit. It's not that I don't want to help her. It's that I'm not even sure I can. I know nothing about sick horses.

"Who else is at the barn?"

As I ask, I'm wrapping a towel around me, heading into my room.

"Nobody, Ellie!" Her voice rises, squeaks; her panic races my own pulse. "It's Monday! The barn is always closed on Monday. That's why Laney wanted me to check on the horses – in case she's really late."

I cross to the window that looks out to the driveway. No cars. No surprise. Both my parents were heading

THROW YOUR HEART OVER

straight from work to Melinda's to go over the seating
plan one more time.

"Ellie? Can you help me?"

"Of course, Sash. I will. I just have to make a phone call
…"

"Don't hang up!" Her voice shrills into my ear.

"OK. Listen, I'm going to put my cell phone down and
make a call on my landline. I won't be able to talk to you
for a couple of minutes, but I'll pick the phone back up as
soon as I can."

I go to my call history. Find the last number that called
me.

*This isn't what he had in mind. This isn't what he bargained
for. I shouldn't ask him.*

But this is Sasha, all alone. This is a horse that needs
help. This is Sasha's horse.

I have to do what I have to do. I punch Terrell's number into the land line receiver and try to remember to
breathe while I listen to his phone ring.

Chapter Twenty-One

"Thank you." I've said it half-a-dozen times since Terrell backed out of my driveway with me in his passenger seat.

In fact, most of what I've said has been "Thank you," and "I'm sorry," only broken up with directions, "Turn left here," or "It's best to take the Queensway."

Terrell keeps saying, "Don't worry," and "It's fine," and "Don't be."

I can't stop myself, though. "I'm sorry."

"I'm not."

His unexpected response earns a new one from me. "Pardon me?"

"I'm absolutely not sorry. I'm happy to be taking you."

"But, dinner."

"We'll eat later."

"I don't know how long it's going to take."

"It doesn't matter."

It doesn't matter. I roll the words around in my head. I love them. They make me want to thank him. Except I've already kind of done that one to the point of meaninglessness.

I try something different. "OK, then I'm not sorry either," and I know I've gotten it exactly right when the light from outside glints off his full-toothed smile.

***

Most of the rest of the drive is spent on the phone.

Sasha calls. "Are you coming?"

"I'm in the car."

"Don't get in an accident."

"My friend's driving. He's a really good driver." I turn to Terrell with my eyebrows lifted. He grins and shoots me a quick thumbs-up before carefully and exaggeratedly replacing his hand on the wheel. "We'll be there soon," I tell her.

"I'm phoning from Laney's office in the main barn. That's how I got your number. But I'm going back to the small barn so come right there, OK?"

"I will, Sash. Twenty minutes."

"OK."

Her voice is tiny and shaky, and I think of all the things she's taught me, and all the things she's talked me through, and even if I'm totally useless in every other way, I want to hug her.

I wasn't lying. Terrell is a careful and steady driver. He's taken that worry away from me.

Watching him check his mirrors, indicate his lane changes, makes me think of me driving and Em watching me. Which makes me think of Em. Which is the most brilliant idea I've had so far.

I gasp, and grab for my phone.

"You OK?" Terrell asks.

"Better than OK. You've just given me the best idea ever."

He shrugs and laughs. "Sure. If you say so."

I've already tried Laney, twice, but Em ... *perfect*.

I scroll for her name and she answers in full flight. "I knew you'd call me for advice on what to wear for your big date. Definitely your skinny jeans – the ones you think are too tight, but they're not, Ellie, they make your butt look great ..."

I shoot a look at Terrell, wonder if he can hear her. "Em ..."

"... and the black turtleneck sweater that shrunk in the wash so you can actually see you have breasts ..."

I hope he can't.

"Em!" My raised voice makes her hesitate, and into the pause I say, "What's colic?"

The sharp intake of her breath, and the too-high pitch of her voice when she gasps, "Is it Lucas?" tell me it's not good.

"It's Oreo," I say, and explain Sasha's phone call.

The more familiar, calm and rational version of Em tells me colic is both "very common" and "possibly very serious."

"Shouldn't a vet be going instead of me?" I ask her. "Is there even anything I can do when I get there?"

"Give me a minute. I can find the vet's number and I'll ask her to meet you there. I'll also ask her what she wants you to do in the meantime. I'll call you back."

I guide Terrell off the highway at the proper exit and peer ahead into the dark through the rain slashing and the wipers swoosh-swooshing across the windshield.

The phone rings in my hand with Em's name on the screen. "OK, Ellie, the vet's going to meet you there and I'm texting you some instructions for colic care."

"What if I don't understand them?"

"Show them to Sasha. The two of you can figure them out – it's nothing that complicated."

"OK, Em. Thanks."

"And, Ellie?"

"Yes?"

"What about your dinner?"

I clear my throat. "Um, Terrell's driving me."

"Terrell's driving you where? To dinner later?"

"I am sitting in the passenger seat of Terrell's car, and he is driving me to the barn."

THROW YOUR HEART OVER

Em lets out a whoop so loud it makes me yank the phone away from my ear.

The corner of Terrell's mouth is twitching. "I don't suppose there's any way you didn't hear that?" I ask.

"Hear what?" But he's full-on grinning now.

I lift the phone back to my ear. "And on that subtle note, I'm going to say good-bye. I'll let you know how Oreo is."

***

Terrell is a champion. He keeps me calm, which lets me calm Sasha down.

When I ask him to hold Oreo's head he says, "I've never touched a horse before," and I say, "Could you do it anyway?" and he nods and says, "Show me," and I move him into position in front of the very obviously sick pony.

The temperature's plunged so low that I'm expecting the rain to morph to snow any minute, but Oreo's sweating. And bumping his nose at his sides. And, when he's not doing that, he's just generally drooping. Tail, ears, head, neck – all have a dejected downward trajectory.

It's clear in no-seconds-flat that take-charge Sasha is totally off-kilter and not taking charge of anything. I run back over Em's instructions in my head.

"Take all the food and water out of his stall," I tell Sasha. She does it. Apparently she'll respond to orders – she just can't make decisions on her own.

"And let's get him a blanket."

"But he's sweating!"

"Which will make him even colder if he's not covered up."

She brings a wool rug which we throw over his back.

"I think we're supposed to walk him, but it's *pouring*," she says. "We can't take him out in that."

"It's all good," I say. "Find me a towel." While she's doing that, I re-check Em's last text message. When Sasha gets back I say, "OK, you stand on that side of him, and pass the towel underneath him to me. Now, do you have a good grip? Lift and hold it snug against his belly until I tell you to stop."

I count to fifteen in my head. Slowly. "Stop!" I tell her. Count to fifteen and say, "Again!"

Soon Terrell takes over the counting, and there's a weird camaraderie in the dim stall with the rain pelting against the window with a noise that suggests it's turning to sleet, and the body heat we're all generating keeping the temperature tolerably warm.

In fact, it's quite jarring when the barn door swings open and the vet stomps in, bringing a spray of rain and an eddy of cold air, but I'm instantly glad to see her.

She comes into the stall and begins examining Oreo and says, "Now tell me what you've been doing ..." and

Laney appears right on her heels saying, "When I read your texts I bullied a police officer into driving me home."

I lead Terrell to Laney's office in the main barn where we make hot drinks for everybody, and by the time we get back Sasha's jumping up and down. "He pooped! He pooped!"

Which, apparently, means Oreo is probably going to be OK, although the vet's giving Sasha a long list of recommendations and things to look out for. "Don't worry – I'm going to sleep in the barn with him tonight," she says.

It also means Terrell and I can make our way home.

The car's cold at first, and I have an odd feeling of being cast out from the warmth and intensity of Oreo's stall. It suddenly seems crazy that I called a guy I just met to drive me into the middle of the country in the dark, in a rain-verging-on-snow storm, to try to treat an equine condition I have no expertise at all with.

But I did. We did.

We're both quiet while Terrell navigates the car through the driving rain, around and through potholes. Once he merges onto the highway he flexes his fingers, settles them back around the steering wheel, and says, "That horse, taking care of him, the things you did ... I had no idea."

"Yeah," I say. "You know what? Neither did I."

He laughs, and I laugh, and the car's nice and warm now, and my stomach gives a massive and very not-delicate, not-classy, not-sexy grumble and I throw my hands across it and say, "I guess I'm hungry."

"How do you feel about the diner?" he asks.

"I love the diner."

"Because it's not very fancy, and I was planning something a little nicer, but it's kind of late, and ..."

"Terrell?"

"Yes?"

"Remember how I kept saying I was sorry earlier?"

"Um ... yeah ..."

"I want to go to the diner."

He grins. "OK. We're going to the diner."

"Excellent. Now let me call Em and tell her how we saved Oreo's life – or at least made him poop – then we can eat."

Chapter
Twenty-Two

The diner was a good choice.

It's comfortable in every way – from the deep booths with their cushy seats, to the not-too-bright-not-too-dim lighting (including no pot lights to serve as downward-pointing spotlights on my face), to the fact that I always know that alongside the classic burgers and club sandwiches, they'll have something I'll love eating, like the black-bean-corn-salsa-spinach-and-a-bunch-of-other-stuff bowl I'm digging into now.

Terrell's eating a breakfast club, obviously assembled from scratch, from the actual yolk oozing out of the sandwich, to the hand cut fries.

And we're both having milkshakes, because you have to at the diner.

We're quiet for the first few minutes after the food arrives. I hadn't realized how hungry I was.

With half his sandwich gone, Terrell leans back and says, "OK, guess I should take a break before I inhale the whole thing without tasting it."

"Yeah, I'm sorry we had to eat so late, especially the night before you're leaving – you probably wanted to be home by now so you could get ready."

"Actually, there are about twenty women at my house right now, and I'm not sure who's happier I'm not there: me, or them. Eating now means if I'm lucky they'll be wrapping up when I get home."

I lift my eyebrows.

"Baby shower for my older sister." He explains. "I told you the hoopla around baby number one was crazy, and it doesn't seem to be easing off for her second one. Although, I have to admit my niece is adorable, and I'm sure I'll feel the same way about her little brother or sister."

"Do you have a picture?"

He thumbs around on his phone and holds it out for me. There's a picture of a very pretty woman squinting into the sun, freckles smattering her pale skin, strands of strawberry-blonde hair blowing across her face, with a curly-haired little girl on her lap waving at the camera. The girl looks like a near-exact miniature of the woman. Neither of them looks anything like Terrell with his smooth deep brown skin, eyes a shade darker, and hair perfectly black.

"I'm adopted," he says.

"I ... oh ..." Funny how my parents have prepared me for a million different scenarios – how to handle them

properly, how to be polite – but never for this one in particular. What is the right thing to say when somebody
tells you they're adopted?

I decide to tell the truth. "I'd be interested in knowing
more about that if you ever want to tell me."

He laughs. "That's not the reaction I normally get."

"Well, I was actually going to say your niece is incredibly cute, and your sister has a great smile, but then you
hijacked the conversation with the whole 'I'm adopted,'
thing."

"I do like to hog the limelight that way, all 'I'm
adopted,' here and 'I'm adopted,' there. I pretty much tell
everyone I can. I'm surprised it took me this long to tell
you."

I shrug. "Lucas did warn me. Said I'd get bored of the
topic."

He sits back against the back of his bench, and I sit
back against mine and we stare at each other with big
smiles on our faces and it's this magical moment that
goes on and on with no awkwardness at all, and I've never
felt anything like it before ...

... and somebody stops dead in front of our booth and
says, "Ellie?"

Oh no.

"Oh my God ... Ellie! I hardly recognized you!"

Her name is Jade. We had grade twelve Biology together. We partnered on a lab. I liked her; she never let on that she noticed my skin when it was bad, but from the way her eyes move from my forehead to my chin, then from one cheekbone to the other, she's obviously noticing the difference now.

"Jade. Hi. Nice to see you. This is my friend, Terrell."

Jade glances at Terrell and tosses him a quick "Hi" before turning back to me.

"You look amazing!" Of course it's so well-intentioned, and meant to be kind, and complimentary, and make me feel good. And it's not her fault that it's the very last thing I want to hear right now – and I especially don't want Terrell to hear it.

Everything in me is tightening – fists, jaw; I'm sure the cords in my neck are standing out – and I want to run away, or to yell at her to shut up, and I know neither of those is the way to handle this. Instead, with a huge effort, I smile. "So do you!"

"Oh, but not like you ..."

I absolutely can't handle it if she gets more specific. Drills down. Says, *I meant your skin – it's so great!*

It's only when a voice calls from the front of the diner, "Jade! Come on – we're not waiting all night!" and she mutters, "Sorry. My *mother*," that I exhale, and realize it's been a while since my last breath.

"You'd better not keep her waiting," I say. "But it was great to run into you."

She gives a little wave and, over her shoulder as she walks away, adds, "You do look fantastic."

When I pull my eyes away from her retreating back and focus back on Terrell he says, "Well, that was ... effusive."

"Good word," I say.

"Seriously, is she like that with everyone, or does she have a crush on you?"

I shrug. "She's just extremely positive."

"If you say so. That seemed a bit ... unusual to me."

I think of how quickly and easily he told me, 'I'm adopted,' when presenting me with the family picture that could have confused me. Surely this is my moment to say, 'I used to have really bad skin. She hasn't seen me since it cleared up.'

The difference is, being adopted is nothing to be embarrassed about. I'm still embarrassed about my skin, and the "bad" phase of it is so recent, I'm still not a hundred per cent confident it's in the past for good. I'm just not ready to talk about it.

Instead I throw the very-sweet Jade under the bus, and say, "Well, maybe she is a bit socially awkward," and a pit of guilt instantly lodges in my stomach that I'm going to have to carry around for the rest of the evening.

***

The rest of the dinner is nice – perfectly fine – nothing wrong with it. It just lacks the magic of earlier. At least I feel like it does.

When the waitress asks if we want dessert I say, "No thanks. Not me, anyway." Terrell nods. "If she's done, then I'm done, too."

We're leaving the diner, shrugging into coats, snugging scarves, pulling on mittens. I have my hand on the door, when I notice a little booth I've always loved the look of, but never sat in – it's empty.

It's tucked in this odd-shaped nook beside the door, enclosed by the front window, and the wall of the store next-door. There's no overhead light, so at this time of night it's dim. It looks cozy, and romantic – which would be the reason I've never sat there – and, all of a sudden I think *Why not?*

I look at Terrell.

I want to sit in there with him.

I take a deep breath.

I need to tell him the truth.

"Ellie?" He's standing behind me, bundled against the cold, probably starting to sweat, probably thinking I've lost my mind.

I turn to face him – turn my back to the door – and say, "Do you think we could stay, and we could order dessert after all, and we could sit there?"

His forehead creases, his eyebrows pull in, he hesitates, then everything clears and he says, "Yes, sure. Of course."

The waitress is walking by and I say, "Actually, I think we've changed our minds. Could you please bring us dessert menus after all, and could we sit there?"

If she raises her eyebrows, or says, "*Oh ... um ... OK ...*" I'll say, "Forget it. Dumb idea." and bolt.

She doesn't though. She winks and says, "Isn't that the best booth?" Then, "I'll bring you menus, but I'll also tell you we have one super-sized peanut-butter brownie left, and if I put some ice cream on the side it would be perfect for sharing."

"Yes," Terrell says. "We'll take that."

So we're staying.

Now I'm nervous.

The re-shedding of our warm layers takes a while, so that's fine, but soon we're sitting in the tiny, intimate booth and Terrell is leaning forward and saying, "What gives?"

What do you mean? It's what I want to say. It's the easy way out. But I already backtracked us to this booth, so I'm committed. Right?

I close my eyes and remember him showing me the picture on his phone. Remember him saying, up-front-and-open, "I'm adopted." Remember how it felt that he shared that with me.

Then I remember how I nearly didn't run with him. How I let my uncertainty fizzle things out after the great time we had running together. How, just now, I killed the easiness of our conversation.

Is my secret serving me well?

Not really.

I dig my phone out of the pocket of my coat. "I have to show you a picture."

It's so stupid that I have a lump in my throat as I scroll for the picture but, there it is; I can hardly swallow. The waitress slides our dessert onto our table and it does look amazingly delicious and, right now, I know there's no way I could force any of it down.

Terrell thanks her for both of us, and I give a weak nod, because I've found the photo.

It was during the period when I'd imposed an almost one-hundred per cent moratorium on anyone taking any photos of me at all, except ... on this particular day not only had our ringette team won a very hard-fought tournament, but I'd played really, really well and I'd been named MVP.

My parents had wanted a picture of me with my medal around my neck and I'd given in. I thought some day I might want to look back on it and, of course, I've never been able to look at it since.

I select it, look just long enough to see it fill the screen, then hand it over to Terrell. "There."

He looks at the screen, then looks up at me. "I ..." He shakes his head. "I want to say 'congratulations' but I feel like that's not what you're getting at by showing me this."

I instinctively lean in to zoom in on my face. To show him *there* where a red lump flames on my cheekbone, and *there* where my temple is so lumpy with cysts I can almost feel the pain of it now.

As I'm moving forward my eyes catch his. I pause. He breathes. It reminds me to breathe.

OK. Stay calm. This isn't show and tell. Just talk to him.

I do. I look him straight on and start: "I'm taking a medication called Acnegon. You might have heard of it. It's pretty much what it says – it's a really strong way to fight acne."

While I'm going, I want to keep going, so I don't pause. Don't really breathe.

"I had really bad acne. I had it until really recently. To be honest, I'm still getting used to my skin being clear, and I'm still pretty self-conscious, and I'm sort of terri-fied it will come back."

I stop, mostly because of the onset of the stinging sensation that warns me tears are imminent. I don't want to cry.

"Oh, Ellie." He's put the phone down. He's holding my hands in his. "I'm sorry that happened to you."

Oh, great. Thanks a lot. The concern in his voice, the sweetness of his response. I sniff once, twice, then make a hiccupping sob noise. "I c-c-can't handle you being so n-n-nice ..."

"Ellie, I'm not being nice. I'm just telling you the truth. Obviously it was – *is* – really upsetting for you."

I nod. "It was hard. I lost my entire social life – except for hanging out with Em and Lucas. I really didn't go anywhere except to school and ringette practice."

"And so ... that girl before?" Terrell tilts his head.

"Yeah, she was surprised because the last time she saw me, my acne was at its worst. I should have just explained it then, and I didn't, and instead I let you think she was the weird one ... I'm sorry." Then, in a small burst of bravery, I whisper. "I only did it because I really like you."

He lifts his hand, reaches toward my cheek, then pauses. "Is this OK?" When I nod, he wipes at a stray tear. "I mean, as reasons go, I guess you liking me is acceptable. Except ..." He sits back. "In the future, how about you just tell me stuff?"

In the future ... "So, you're OK with it?"

He laughs. "I'm actually kind of relieved. I like you so much, but every now and then you'd go weird on me – your sister saying you were painting your toenails, or this sudden stiffness – and I had no idea what it was all about. I mean, don't get me wrong – I think you're beautiful, but I kept wondering, 'Is there something I'm going to find out that I'm going to regret?' This ..." He points at the now-dark phone. "... is nothing."

He lifts his eyes, points to them. "Look at me."

I do.

"Ellie, I sincerely hope your skin stays clear from here on forward – really mostly for your own sake – but if it doesn't, we'll deal with it. OK?"

"OK."

"Now, I like my ice cream a bit soft, but if we wait any longer it's going to be soup, so are you good if we eat this dessert?"

***

When Terrell pulls into my driveway it's still empty of cars. Other than the front porch light, and the lamps on strategically placed timers, the house is dark.

"So, um, good-night," he says.

"Yeah. Thanks for ... well ... everything. The drive, and the help, and the moral support, and dinner. I owe you gas and food."

"You don't owe me anything. It was great."

"You were great ... with Oreo, I mean. You've got the touch." *Shit, did I just say that? Cringe ...*

He's not cringing, though, he's shifted in his seat and he's closer to me. Just like that it's warm in the car and, even though I should be reaching for the door handle, I'm turning toward him.

We're really close, and looking at each other, and it's like that moment in the booth, except this time it's inches instead of feet, and a table separating us.

He clears his throat, and I clear mine, then I run my tongue quickly across my teeth – *spinach, what if there's spinach there?* – then it doesn't matter because his lips are on mine and they're so, so soft and my head's floating while everything else in me is spiraling inward, tightening my core, sparking a longing in me I haven't felt before. It makes me want to climb over the centre console – why do those things have to be so big and clunky? – and press as much of my body against his as I can.

I push back with my lips, and the kiss isn't soft anymore – it's urgent, and now my tongue's running across his teeth, and they're just as smooth as they look when he smiles. We're bumping noses, and it doesn't matter. I'm finding out there's stubble on his cheeks, and I don't care.

He makes a funny noise – kind of a whimper-sigh – and it kills me when he pulls back, because that noise makes me want to kiss him even more. He pushes his forehead against mine and his breath is warm on my face when he says, "Oh, wow, Ellie ..."

I reach up and place my hand in the crook where his neck meets his jaw – where his skin is warm and his pulse is thumping – and he leans his head back. A wash of light from the street lamp spills over his face, highlights all the beautiful contours of his brow, and nose. I can't believe I get to kiss him.

Unfortunately, the street light also illuminates my elderly neighbour taking his slow-shuffling English bulldog, Winston, for his late-evening walk.

Terrell sees them too.

"I guess that's my signal to preserve your good reputation, and get myself to bed before we leave tomorrow."

"Tomorrow ..." I sigh.

He leans toward me again, props his forehead against mine one more time, and says, "I don't even mind going away so much now that I know we've figured this out. It just means we have lots to look forward to after."

Outside Winston barks at a squirrel, or a shadow, or maybe the two of us in the car. "OK, OK," Terrell says. "I'm going ... but I'm just going to put it out there that our bus leaves at 10:00 from the Athletic Centre."

"Hmm ..." I say. "Noted, even though I have no idea why you'd mention that, and I'm sure I'll forget it right away."

He grins. "That's what I thought. Good-night, Ellie."

"Good-night, Terrell."

Chapter
Twenty-Three

In the morning I go to the Athletic Centre to watch the bus pull out. It's one of those big coaches with tinted windows so I have no idea who's on it and who isn't. Until Terrell appears in the door and bounds across the sidewalk to me. "You showed up!"

Him being happy makes me happy. I grin, before dropping my eyes and shaking my head. "Well ... I have class in the Arts building, so ..."

He bends low, straining to catch my downcast gaze. "Really? So you just happened to be walking by?" He claps his hand to his chest. "That hurts."

I give in. Lift my smiling face to him again. "I do have class there, but I'm already ten minutes late."

"Well, girl, you must like me if you're willing to miss ten minutes of class for me."

"It'll be more like fifteen by the time I get there."

"A quarter-of-an-hour. Be still my beating heart."

"I do," I say.

"Do what?"

"Do like you."

"More than last night?"

"Even more than that."

"Well, in that case ..." He leans in and I'm pretty sure he's aiming for my cheek, but at the last second I turn my face into his and it's our lips that connect.

Brief, glancing, but it was a kiss-on-the-lips.

Which is quite enough considering the banging on the bus windows.

He must want to get away now. I've probably just completely embarrassed him.

But he laughs, and sends a dismissive wave toward the bus, and whispers, "Four sleeps."

"Four?" My heart's sinking, and I'm trying not to let it come through in my voice.

"Yeah. Four. Is that a problem?"

I force a smile onto my face. "Only my own problem. On my way over here I finally got up the guts to ask you to my sister's wedding, like I should have way back, and I know I left it too late, and I know it's not your fault, but I was still just kind of ..." I lift my fingers in front of his face where he can see I have them crossed, "... *hoping*. But it's OK. I understand. It's on me ..."

"Ellie?"

"Yes?"

"I really, really, really would like to come to your sister's wedding." He grins, places one of his hands over his heart and gives it a double-thump. "Like, *really*. Coach made us all pack dress pants and a button-down shirt for an alumni dinner we're going to, and if I find out there's any way at all I can make it to the wedding, I'll be there and I won't even have to wear my basketball uniform."

I shrug. "I mean, I do like you in your basketball uniform ... but you'd probably upstage the groom."

"I'll try," he says. "OK?"

I nod. "Definitely. OK." I take a deep breath. "You have to get on the bus."

"And you have to go to your class."

Neither of us moves.

"Oh!" I say. "Is that your coach in the doorway?"

"Whoops. Yes. OK." He goes a few feet before turning around. "I'll text you."

Then he's gone, up the stairs, behind the tinted bus windows.

And that's when I know how much I'm going to miss him.

***

As soon as I get home from school, the phone rings. I answer to hear Melinda's voice at the other end of the line talking to somebody else. "No, it's not *eight* tables of *sixteen,* it's *sixteen* tables of *eight* – who ever heard of a table for sixteen people?"

"Melinda?"

"Those chairs are going to be covered, right? Because ..."

"Melinda!"

"What? Sorry, my sister is talking to me ... yes, Ellie, is that you?"

"You called here, Melinda."

"Yes, well, I need you to go out for me."

"Out, where?"

"Out to Party Central. They ordered my napkins in Iris, when they were clearly supposed to be Heather."

"Iris? Heather?"

"*Colours,* Ellie. Focus. The Iris is all wrong – it'll clash with the table centrepiece. The venue needs the napkins ASAP and the only Party Central with the Heather napkins in stock is the one at the other end of the city from the venue, and there's no way I have time to go there tonight."

"But *I* do, of course."

"Great! I would get you to bring them by the venue, but they'll be closed by the time you get back, so I guess you'll just have to bring them to our place."

While I'm scarfing down dinner, and driving to Party Central, then to Melinda's, I'm alternating between thinking really great, amazing things about Terrell – picturing his smile, reminding myself *he likes me, too,* and then going completely off-track reliving last night's kiss – and kicking myself for not asking him to the wedding sooner.

Not that it would have made a difference. I mean, if he's not back, he's not back.

But at least it wouldn't have felt so rushed.

At least he would have known how I felt about him sooner.

At least, maybe, possibly, there might have been a way we could have made some kind of plan.

Maybe there still is.

Maybe there will be an opportunity I can seize.

Maybe.

"You'd just better be ready to seize it if it comes," I tell myself, then give a great big smile to the guy staring at me from the car at the red light next to me.

He blinks and I throw in a wave. There. Now if I can just be that brave if I have a chance to make it count.

Chapter
Twenty-Four

There's a strangeness about this whole week. It's the countdown to Melinda's wedding and how hard to believe that we're nearly, almost there. It's the equally hard-to-believe fact that Terrell is ... my boyfriend? But probably not my wedding date ... And, punctuating it all is the fact that, instead of getting up and running, and eating breakfast, and going to campus this morning, I'm going completely the opposite direction, out to Lucas, and Laney, and a weekday riding lesson to make up for the one I'm going to miss on Saturday because of the wedding.

It's strange, but also freeing. I'm merging onto the highway. I'm indicating and accelerating, and there's an open spot in traffic just for me and ... I'm going.

It's early – still rush hour – and the cars are bumper-to-bumper the other direction. Heading into town, into school, work, obligations.

Not like me. I'm going to the country.

When a quick flick through the pre-programmed radio stations brings up nothing but ads for car dealerships, and internet services, and paid messages from local candidates in the upcoming election, I find a country station, and lyrics about lying in the back of a pick-up truck, under a summer sky, running barefoot in a rainstorm, speed my transition from city / university / public-transit-riding Ellie, to paddock-boot-wearing, horseback-riding, singing-along-to-Young-Country Ellie.

This new Ellie learns something new with every trip to the barn.

This version of me doesn't let thoughts of past hurts or anxieties, or Melinda's wedding chaos, or my love-life follow me to see Lucas.

Equestrian Ellie's biggest worry is whether I've set my saddle in the right spot on Lucas's back.

As I drive, traffic drops away. Out by the exit for the barn, the only other vehicles on the highway have dealership stickers from Kingston, Sudbury, Toronto. This is a no-man's land where ninety-five per cent of drivers are just passing through.

Not me.

I take the swooping ramp where, last Saturday, a deer leapt across the road right in front of me.

I pass now-familiar paddocks with now-familiar horses. A golf course. A catholic school stuck in the middle of farmers' fields. Kids wing through the air on swings just metres from a wire fence holding back a herd of Holsteins.

And up ahead is the driveway. I slow, then slow more. You can never drive slowly enough around horses.

I'm used to it being quiet when I arrive early on Saturday mornings, but today not even Sasha's here.

She emailed me last night, as she has been every night, sending updates on Oreo's continuing miraculous recovery. **I wish I could be there for your make-up lesson in the morning, but my mom won't let me skip school. At least I'll see you on Saturday. I'm so excited! By the way, the dress fits perfectly …**

It's amazing how quickly it's become second nature to walk to Lucas's small barn.

I'm a little worried. What if he's not in? I think I know where to find him, and I'm pretty sure I could get him, and it would probably be OK, but … I step into the barn and there's a snort and a rustle, and Lucas's head pops over the stall door.

Oh! He's in. And … does he know me? It seems like he knows me. He's definitely poking his nose toward me and he's making a kind of rumbling noise. "Hey you," I say. "Is that how you say hi?"

I lift the halter off the hook on the front of his stall. "OK, let's see if I know what I'm doing."

After my initial flurry of nerves I settle into the rhythm I've learned – hooves, different brushes, tail (it was one of Em's conditions for me riding him; "For the love of God, please keep my filthy horse's tail clean), saddle pad, then gel pad, and saddle.

Do up the girth, but not too tight. Put the stirrups to hole number seven.

I've done it automatically. Haven't second-guessed myself. Until Laney pokes her head in the door. "Ready?"

"Um ... I think so?"

"Well, let's double-check, shall we?"

***

It's all good. "Very good," Laney says.

"It's thanks to Sasha," I say.

Laney smiles. "Sasha's a good teacher, and you're a quick learner."

We'll see about that.

Laney wants me to jump. "At the end of the lesson. After we ride over some trot poles. Just one, little jump.

It's not that I'm against the idea, it's that the idea is nearly unfathomable. "I never thought I'd be jumping."

"What did you think you'd be doing?"

"Honestly?" I shrug. "I guess I thought I'd be riding for eight weeks. I figured I'd use it to get me through my sister's wedding ..." I hesitate, and look sideways at Laney "... and not being able to play ringette anymore, and not really knowing how to go about having a social life in university ... and then, you know, the program would be over, and I'd be past those things – or at least used to them – and that would be it."

"Do you still think that?"

A breeze ruffles Lucas's mane. A horse whinnies in the distance. Up so high it can't touch, or affect me, a vapour trail wisps away in the bright autumn sky.

Lucas reaches for the bit, and I've learned to hold my hands steady because doing so will let him connect with me.

"No," I say. *How could it?* I don't say that part, but I think Laney gets it.

She nods. She smiles. "I didn't think so. Not after your adventures with Oreo the other night. I have something to talk to you about."

"What?"

"Later," she says. "First Operation Throw Your Heart Over."

"Pardon me?"

"I'll explain more later."

***

I nearly give up at the trot pole stage. "Um ..."

"Yes? Is there a problem?"

"No. Not one. Three, that I can identify off the top of my head."

"Which are?"

I resist the urge to pull on Lucas's mouth to make him stop. Sasha taught me early on that it's only in the movies that people yank on the reins and yell, "Whoa!" Or, at least, it *should* only be in the movies.

Instead I close my fingers on the reins, stop moving my hips, straighten my back, and Lucas walks, then halts.

I drop the reins and count off using my fingers. "One, we're ridiculously wobbly. Two, he hits some of the poles, and jumps over other ones. Three, he slows down and speeds up." I shake my head. "Basically, we're a hot mess."

Laney nods. "Yes, well, recognition is the first step to improvement and, lucky for you, all three issues can be helped by the same thing."

Impulsion.

It's a word I doubt I've ever heard before – I certainly can't remember it ever dropping into casual conversation.

Laney tells me it's, "Going forward with controlled power." then adds, "I stole the definition from Wikipedia."

I've always felt like I was lucky. I've watched a couple of the other kids in the learn-to-ride program. Watched how Laney had to chase their ponies around the ring to make them trot. Watched them drop boldly back to a "I-don't-really-care-if-you-want-to-go-faster" walk the minute she stopped running after them.

"Lucas goes," I tell Laney.

Her lifted eyebrows prompt me to mentally review the definition. "Go" is a small part of it. There's also "forward" and "with controlled power."

OK, so up until now, Lucas going truly has been all about luck. He likes to go, so he goes. I have no power, or control over it. I just happily post along in the trot.

"Fine," I sigh. "Talk to me about the controlled power ..."

***

By the end of the lesson, I get it.

Or, at least I'm sort-of, somewhere-on-the-path to getting it, and Lucas and I have maybe actually, truly achieved it once or twice for a few blissful seconds.

We do one set of trot poles where he – I swear – floats over them. "Can you feel that?" Laney asks, and I'm already nodding so hard I think my head might fall off. *Is she kidding?* How could I *not* feel it? It was heavenly.

Of course, it only makes the next, quite terrible set seem even worse. "Ugh!" I yell as Lucas knocks, and bumps, and swerves his way through them.

Still, we manage two more very nice (even if not completely floaty) trips through the poles and Laney says, "That's it. Time to jump."

The jump, I realize, is not big. I mean, I could jump over it myself, with no effort at all, and it will be so much easier for Lucas.

I squint my eyes at the criss-crossed poles. "I don't think it's the jump itself," I tell Laney. "It's that I don't want to do one of those jerky bump-around things over it like I did with the trot poles. Only, I assume it would feel worse with an actual jump."

"Well," Laney says. "That is, actually, preventable. We need to go back to the thing I said earlier; the thing about throwing your heart over."

"I'm listening."

"There's this saying in jumping – 'Throw your heart over, then jump over after it.' Does that make any sense to you?"

Those words – they don't travel to my brain – instead they pierce my heart.

There are things in life guaranteed to overwhelm me with emotion: holding a kitten, fireworks on Canada Day, footage of Terry Fox. Or Gord Downie. Listening to the lyrics of pretty much any song by The Killers. The first snowfall of the year.

Throw your heart over. Just like those other things on my list, something about those words hits me so hard that it hurts, but I also want to keep feeling it.

If the idea's that good, I've got to see what the actual jump feels like. I gather my reins. "Let's go."

"All the hard work was in the trot poles," Laney says. "The jump really won't be anything big, or dramatic, just keep doing what you've been doing."

I send Lucas into a trot, and it's nice and forward, and straight, and even – I'd even argue it has impulsion to it – and it only gets scary when we leave the circle and are on the straight line which clearly means we're only going to do one thing, and it's that jump. I get ready to hold his mane if I have to, and don't even let myself think of circling away. I just take a really deep breath and puff my chest out and *throw my heart over* and we both jump over after it.

The jump is easy, and I wonder if it was all too easy, then Lucas flicks one ear back and gives a little bumpety kick, just to make my heart skip a couple of beats and Laney laughs and says, "He feels good!"

I ride him in a really big, as-round-as-I-can-make-it circle and Laney says, "Great job! Scratch his withers."

"What did you think?"

"It was fun ..."

"There's a 'but' in there."

I shrug. "I mean, I guess, I wouldn't mind ..."

"... jumping higher?" Laney gives a fist pump. "I knew it!"

Laney nudges the jump up one hole on each side, and the angles of the X sharpen. Lucas and I do it again much like the first time: *impulsion, impulsion, impulsion, throw heart, hop, catch up to heart.*

Then again – a steeper X.

The final time, Laney puts the bar straight across.

OK. That suddenly looks quite a bit larger.

Which is when I realize I may, perhaps, not have been throwing my *entire* heart over.

I guess it's time to start now.

Trot. Forward, with contact. Circle round. Approach straight.

It's big ...

It doesn't matter.

Not if I do what I have to do.

I keep my eyes wide open, take a deep, deep breath, and send my heart hurtling out in front of me.

Lucas jumps up under me, and this time it's different. This time we catch up with my heart in mid-air and it's in my chest, lifting me up, and I land smiling.

***

Lucas's tack is clean, and so is he, I've turned him out to enjoy the gorgeous fall sunshine with his equine friends, and I'm sweeping the aisle of the small barn when Laney comes to find me.

"So," she says. "Those things I wanted to talk to you about – do you have a few minutes now?"

"Sure – I really just need to get back in time for a quick shower before I head to campus for my afternoon class. I'm trying to minimize my time spent at home these days because my sister's gotten into the habit of leaving messages there with last-minute wedding errands to do."

"About that," Laney says. "The wedding I mean – it's so nice of you to involve Sasha. She's beyond excited."

I shrug. "I like her. And it was starting to look like I wouldn't have anyone to bring to the wedding, anyway, so ..."

Laney's eyebrows shoot up. "What about that guy who drove you out here the other night when Oreo was colicking? The one so tall he hardly fit in the stall? Oreo liked him."

Laney's tone is clear. The horse liked him. He's good people.

She gives me a closer look. "Are you blushing?"

I laugh. "Yeah, I might be. Both because, you're right, he's amazing, and also because he's out of town on a basketball tour this weekend, so ..." I shrug.

"How far out of town?"

"Pardon me?"

"Well, I wouldn't say this around any of the younger kids ..." She looks left, then right, as though there might be small riders lurking in the shadows of the aisle, "... but there was a time I got my horse bedded down in his show stabling at the Royal, slipped a groom twenty dollars to do extra checks on him, and drove two hours north to ... well ..." More furtive glances. "... to *meet* somebody."

I open my eyes as wide as they'll go. "Oh? Like meet your grandma for tea?"

She thwacks at my paddock boot with the crop she's carrying. "I love my grandma, but she's never made my heart jump."

"Oh, so we're talking about a 'Throw Your Heart Over' scenario?"

Laney smiles. "See, I said you were a good student ... speaking of which ... let's talk about my proposal. There are two things, and both of them have to do with you sticking around here for longer than eight weeks. So, will you? Stick around for longer than eight weeks?"

A chunk of hair falls in my face and I brush it away with a grime-encrusted hand that smells like horse. I re-adjust my grip on the broom and a broken blister twinges. I glance down and spot the smear that won't wash out that has made this particular grey hoodie that I'm wearing my riding hoodie.

I wrinkle my nose. "How could I leave?"

Laney smiles. "Just so you know, it's going to get cold around here. There's nothing more bone-chilling than an indoor arena in January. And the manure will freeze into little balls you can break your ankle on."

"And here I thought you were happy to have me around."

"I just don't want you to accuse me of luring you to stay under false pretenses."

"When you say 'stay' what, exactly, do you mean?"

"I wondered if you'd be willing to work here."

"Work? How can I work here? A couple of months ago I'd barely even touched a horse."

She points to the broom I'm leaning on. "Well, right there I see the two main attributes you need to qualify for the job: a) you know how to sweep, and b) you don't think it's beneath you."

Work? Here? My head's spinning.

"Listen," Laney says. "Here's the deal. We always have a spot open for night check or weekend work – essentially I try to find people to do it, and if I can't, I do it, so there's definitely a spot for you. I can give you one shift a week, or more, whatever works for you. You'd work your way through the barns, picking out stalls, feeding, watering, sweeping, and generally doing stuff that needs to be done. You can get paid partially in free lessons, partially in cash – we can work out the details. You don't need to decide now, but tell me soon. Questions?"

Laney's pretty much covered all the practical stuff, so the main questions I'm left with is, *Could I really do this?* The one question I don't have is *Do I want to do this?* The answer to that is a resounding Yes. I like looking after Lucas for free, so the idea of getting paid to do more of the same is amazing.

"Um, no. No questions at this moment. I'll have to look at my schedule and talk to my mom about having the car …"

"Of course. Talk to her, then talk to me. In the meantime we'll talk about the other thing."

Oh, yeah. The other thing. Laney's already shocked me once – what's next?

"A show," she says.

At least, that's what I think she said. Maybe I heard her wrong. "Pardon me?"

"I'm not sure if you remember I said I was running this program in conjunction with another stable – Stonegate? – anyway, they're having their final schooling show of the season in a couple of weeks and they're hoping at least some members of the group will compete."

"Compete?" It's kind of like the jumping – it's not that I'm nervous; it's that I can't even wrap my head around the idea. *Me?* I'm so new to riding I don't even know what a horse competition, or show, or whatever, looks like. The one thing I'm pretty sure of is that it's miles away from a ringette tournament.

"It won't be anything you can't do. I promise. And Lucas has been to Stonegate lots of times – it's no big deal for him – he'll be rock-solid. When they set up the classes for this show, they included a couple of special ones for Learn to Ride students – they'll be small classes; just you guys, and some students from previous sessions, and a few from other programs in the area."

"Stonegate?" I'm comfortable here. I can't imagine going somewhere else – especially not for a competition.

Laney steps forward and puts her arms around me. She pulls me in for a hug, and through my hair I hear the mumble of her voice. "I'm so proud of you, Ellie. You're our star pupil. You have a way with horses. And I know you have a lot going on, so how about we say you just get through your sister's wedding, and put the show in the back of your mind, and you can tell me after?"

Star pupil. It does sound nice.

When I step out of the hug, I say, "I do have one question."

"Which is?"

"Well, you did it. You paid off the groom and drove all that way. And ...?"

She bites her lip and now she's the one blushing. "And, it was worth it."

Chapter Twenty-Five

I make it to campus with half-an-hour to spare.

It gives me time to stop in at the Tim Horton's around the corner from the tables where I sat with Addy, and Olivia, and Sophia, and order two small hot chocolates with whipped cream, because it's cold outside, and I got to ride this morning, and I'm glad Addy's my friend, and she likes hot chocolate. With whipped cream.

Addy's not in class.

Which is weird.

Addy told me she didn't skip one single class in her whole high school career. "I'm not about to start in university," she said. "For me it would be a slippery slope. Miss a class, get behind, get worried, miss the next class, next thing I know I've wasted the tuition my mom cleans houses to pay for."

So why isn't she here today?

I text her. **All OK? Really missing you in class today. I need social contact with somebody I'm not related to.**

No reply at break.

No reply by the end of class.

The only thing I can think of is that Addy's too sick to come, and too sick to text, and the way I was raised, when you're that sick you need someone to check on you.

Unfortunately my mom's not available, so it's going to have to be me.

I text again **Not happy that you're not here + not answering. Going to drop by and check on you.**

The phone vibrates while it's still in my hand.

No. Don't. Please.

Why not?

I'm not fit for contact with outside world.

I know exactly how she feels. Now I'm definitely going.

***

It takes approximately thirty-seven seconds for me to breach the residence security. I mean, granted, I'm a skinny-jean wearing, backpack-toting, first-year student with my hair in a ponytail. I like to think somebody wearing fatigues and holding a weapon would have a harder time getting in, but the girl who holds the door open for me doesn't look at me for even the blink of an eye.

Whatever. I wanted in and I'm in.

Turns out Addy's door is going to be much harder than the entrance doors. It's closed tight, heavy, solid, and she doesn't answer my knock.

I pull out my phone **From your assertion that you're not fit for the outside world, I'm assuming you're in there.**

Ellie. I told you not to come. Go away. She puts a heart at the end. I guess that's a "Please-don't-allow-my-"go-away"-to-hurt-your-feelings emoji.

Nope. Not going away.

There are two truths about this little sit-in / stand-in I'm mounting in Addy's hallway. One is that I'm truly worried about her and I'm not going to relax until I make contact with her.

Two is that I'm trying to channel the brave feeling I have from Laney's encouragement to throw my heart over – two different ways – and trying not to wish I'd been willing to do it sooner.

I'll do it from now on.

Starting now.

An ear-bud-wearing guy walks by without even look-ing at me but I'm not above a bit of lying. **Your floormates are coming by and giving me looks. If you** don't let me in soon, everyone will be speculating about why I'm lurking outside your door.

When that gets no response, I add **I'm going to start making up stories. I'm going to tell them you owe me money.**

Lots of money.

Because I'm your bookie and you lost a bet about what colour Andrew Scheer's boxer shorts are.

The door opens, Addy's hand comes out, she grabs my sleeve and pulls me in.

She stands in front of me, puffy-eyed, cheeks wet with tears, an incredibly painful-looking cyst on the side of her nose, and says, "There. Now you can see why I couldn't leave my room today. Are you happy now?"

I shake my head. "No. Of course I'm not happy. But I'd like to help you if you'll let me."

"No ..." she says. "No, no, no." She's crying, and her nose is running, and it's just making everything worse, but she knows that. The thing is, while she's saying no, she's nodding her head.

I decide to take that as a yes.

I cross the room to her mini-fridge, switch on the kettle sitting on top of it, and say, "I'm going to make us some tea, and we're going to figure this out."

Then I pick up my phone and find Dr. Hamilton's cell number.

**

An hour later Addy, Rachel, and I are standing in the familiar beige-carpeted, -walled, -ceilinged hallway outside Dr. Hamilton's door, listening to the latch being turned.

Dr. Hamilton opens the door herself. "Come on in."

We step into the completely empty waiting room with the reception area dark and the glass hatch closed.

"I'm sorry," I start. "It's after-hours. You should be heading home ..."

She cuts me off. "I told you to come. I'm always happy to see my favourite sisters." She turns to Addy. "And you must be Adeline."

Addy lifts her eyes from the ground long enough to half-nod and Dr. Hamilton says, "Great. You can leave your coat here, then come on into my examination room that's as close to cozy as an examination room can be, and we can talk."

We're all shucking out of coats, and yanking off boots when my phone vibrates.

I take a second to look down at the notification. New message. From Terrell.

Oh. Wow.

I look up, smile at Addy, and think, *I can read it in just a few seconds ...*

"You're coming, right Ellie?"

"Oh, I can wait here so you can have some privacy."

She snorts. "Really? You mean like in my residence hallway?"

The snort is a good sign. It's a glimmer of the usual Addy. I look at Dr. Hamilton and she says, "Of course, if Adeline wants you with her." I look at Rachel and think of how she's been beside me every step of the way.

I shove my phone in my pocket.

"Yes. Of course. My pleasure."

We go in together, and Addy sits where I normally do, and I sit in Rachel's usual chair, and Dr. Hamilton says, "Well, Adeline, I can see that you have severe, scarring acne, and I'd like to help you with that."

Addy turns to me. "Did you feel this good when she said that to you?"

I nod. "They were some of the most beautiful words I'd ever heard."

***

We drop a much-calmer Addy off at the door to her residence. She's clutching a Subway bag to match the ones both Rachel and I have.

The deal we made is that Addy will eat her Subway in her room, hibernate for the rest of the night, then get up in the morning, take a deep breath, and get back to her routine. Oh, and I'm meeting her at the front door of her residence tomorrow morning to walk her to her first class.

"Do you want me to come up with you?" I ask her.

"No. I'm good now. I'll see you in the morning."

Still, Rachel and I sit and watch while she goes through the doors, and we don't stop watching until we see her step onto the elevator.

"Thanks a million, Rach," I say.

"Hey. Thanks for calling me. Seriously. We were going into hour three of a strategic planning meeting and we'd just looped back to the first item on the agenda. I was about to commit murder."

"Glad we could help."

"Do you think she'll be OK?" Rachel asks. This time her voice is serious.

"I think this is the best chance she stands of being OK. I know it's a long road yet. It's so frustrating to have to wait the month before starting the medication, but the clock starts ticking today, so hopefully she'll get some of her usual positive energy back to ride it out."

My phone goes, and my heart jumps. Tell me it's not Addy already up in her room lapsing back to despair.

Rachel's raised eyebrows tell me she's wondering the same thing.

It's not Addy.

I turn to Rachel and mouth "Me-lin-da."

"Shit," she mouths back.

I giggle, and Melinda says, "I'm sorry. Is there something funny about the fact that the store just called to say my table gifts haven't been picked up yet – the table gifts that were clearly assigned to you to pick up?"

"Not at all," I tell her. "I'm on it."

I hang up and Rachel's shaking her head. "No way. We are not doing one single thing before we find a place to park this car and eat these subs."

"Agreed. And while we're at it, I have a message to read."

***

Missing you. Only have a few minutes before going into the gym. Here are the deets I know so far. The Sunday morning game isn't for sure.

I squeal.

"What is it?" Rachel asks around a mouthful of Chicken and Bacon Ranch Melt.

"I promise I'll tell you. In a minute."

Coach has it penciled in but the gym we're supposed to play in might be double-booked. Don't know yet, but you'll know as soon as I do. Gotta go. Did I mention I'm missing you?

"So?" Rachel swipes a glob of mayo from the corner of her mouth and points at my now-blank phone screen. "What?"

"So ..." I say. "That was Terrell."

"And ...?"

I pop a pickle in my mouth, enjoy the salty crunch, and nod, "And, yes."

Rachel punches my arm, steals a pickle, and I'm not even angry, because the smile on her face when she says, "Oh, thank goodness for that!" is definitely just as wide as mine.

Chapter Twenty-Six

Of course, basking in warm fuzziness can only last so long with Rachel around. "Is he coming to the wedding?"

I sigh.

"Ah-ha – I *knew* it!" Rachel crumples up her sub packaging and says, "I'll drive you out to pick up Melinda's table gifts on the condition that you call that boy right now and invite him to the wedding."

"The 'ah-ha's on you, Rach, because I did invite him."

"And?"

"And ... it's complicated."

"Ellie, don't give me that." Her voice is a growl.

I'm tired, and I'm frustrated, and I want Terrell at the wedding, and I've had enough. I growl back. Literally growl. So loudly that my sister pulls back.

"No, Rach. *You* don't give *me* that. I want him to come. I'm going to be sad and lonely if he doesn't come. I've already gone way out of my comfort zone with this guy –

and he's totally worth it – but still, I think I deserve a little credit. If he's not there, it won't be because I didn't try."

She's quiet for a minute, then she puffs out her breath in a forceful exhale, "Wow. Nice one, sis. Are you prepared to put that passion into trying to get him to the wedding?"

"Isn't that what I just said?"

"OK, then you just let me know how I can help."

"Oh," I say. "OK, thanks."

"We good?" she asks.

I nod. "We're good."

She turns the ignition. "OK, let's go get these goddamn table gifts."

***

After the frantic pace we've been keeping up, I don't know how there are still errands to do on the day before the wedding, but there still are. Lots of them.

Everyone meets at my parents' house bright and early and we're divided into teams – it's the closest I've ever felt to being on the Amazing Race – and, fortunately, I'm paired with Paige.

My kind, not-nosy, patient, sweet-tempered sister is the perfect person to make the hectic pre-wedding afternoon bearable.

When we've criss-crossed the city, dropping things off at the venue not once, but twice – having to re-fill the gas tank after all that driving – and we're at our final stop – the department store again, waiting for the final round-up of Melinda's registry items – we lower ourselves onto ugly vinyl-covered chairs and I laugh at the farting noises they make when we sit.

"Stand up again," I urge Paige.

My sister shakes her head. "Honestly, Ellie. I don't know how you have the energy. I am so tired."

What I don't admit is, it's nervous energy. Keep talking, doing, babbling, running. I woke up to a text from Terrell. **No news. Except I still miss you. But that isn't news.** I've Googled every mode of transport known to man, pored over timetables, added up fares, then tried to figure out at what point making a romantic effort crosses the line into behaving like an obsessed person. What seems reasonable one minute, seems impossible the next.

Meaningless chatter is a great defence mechanism against facing possible defeat, and in that spirit, I give Paige a flip reply. "Oh yeah? Why so worn out? Hot night with Nathan?"

When Paige's cheeks flame red I'm hit with instant remorse. I always think my other two sisters are too hard on her, but here I go. "Sorry," I say. "Of course you're tired. We've been running around in circles."

Paige puts her hand on my arm. "No, it's OK."

I look down at her hand, then up at her eyes, and they're brimming with tears. "What is it Paigey?" *Oh no, please tell me Nathan hasn't dumped her right before the wedding.* "What's wrong?"

"Nothing's wrong."

On closer inspection, her eyes are very, very shiny and the trademark smile dimple that makes her the cutest of all us sisters, is showing. "Wait a minute ... are you crying because you're happy?"

Paige bites her lips together and rummages in her purse. After a couple of seconds she brings her hand out and it's adorned with the most delicate ring I've ever seen. On her left ring finger.

"Oh!" I take hold of her hand and lift it. "Is that ...?"

She nods. "It was Nathan's grandmother's. Isn't it beautiful? He asked me last night, and I want to tell the whole world, but it's Melinda's big weekend ..." She looks at me. "You'll keep it a secret, right?"

I blink. Now my eyes have gone blurry. "Of course I will, if you want me to, but this is so exciting! You're the nicest sister in the world for not telling anybody. I'm sure Melinda would be happy for you."

Paige clears her throat and I laugh. "OK, she'll be happy for you *after* she's had her moment in the limelight."

"You know what, Ellie? It doesn't matter anyway. Nathan is so great, it doesn't matter if I have to wait a little while to tell everyone we're engaged." She leans in and we hug, then she adds. "Now I just want you to meet somebody amazing."

I hesitate. Have an internal should-I-shouldn't-I debate that lasts a few seconds, but feels like forever. Then say, "Since we're sharing secrets, actually, there is somebody I like. And he's really nice."

"Oh!" Paige claps her hand. "Is that your mystery wedding guest? The one we've been fighting for Melinda to let you bring?"

I cross my fingers. "I hope so. I really, really hope so."

***

Our house is in chaos.

All my sisters are having dinner at our house, but it's not going to be one of my mom's nice, sit-down meals. At the moment there's a heated debate raging about which dishes of Chinese take-out to order, with the list spilling onto a second sheet.

The whole time, people are dashing to answer the phone, and opening the door to delivery after delivery of congratulatory flower bouquets.

I only notice too late that Paige has forgotten to take off her engagement ring and I'm trying to signal it to her when Rachel spots it which leads to hugging and tears and – thank goodness – good wishes from Melinda who sobs into Paige's hair and says, "I can't wait to be your matron of honour."

When my phone rings I hardly hear it over the din. A quick glance sends my heart hammering. **Terrell.**

I sprint to my room, answering halfway up the stairs. "Hi. It's me. My house is crazy. I'm going to my room so I can hear you."

Inside, I turn my back to my door, and gasp. "I'm here. It's quiet. I've been dying to hear from you."

"Oh," he says.

"Oh what?"

"Oh, hearing your voice makes me really, really want to come home for that wedding."

My stomach drops. "That sounds to me like you can't."

"Well, the Sunday game is off."

Even as my heart is lifting, jumping, flying, he's saying, "But, wait, Ellie. I've been so focused on that, I haven't even been thinking about Saturday. The guys play in Kingston at noon ..."

"That's OK!" I break in. I should know. I've been doing so many calculations over the last couple of days that these come to me automatically now. Game at noon, finishes around 1:30, which should get their bus home around 3:30, which means he might miss part of the ceremony ... which would be a shame ... but he'd be there for most everything.

"No, wait, Ellie. The girls' game is after."

"Oh." Of course. That pushes everything back. "I should have known that. I don't know what I was thinking."

"You were doing what I've been doing – wishful thinking."

I sigh. "You're right."

There are voices, noises in the background of his call. "Listen, Ellie, we have a game in fifteen minutes. I should be warming up. I'll text you later. I'll tell you if anything changes."

"Go play! Have fun!" I force my voice to be happy, cheerful. I want him to hang up on a high note.

With the call over, in the quiet of my room, I have a decision to make.

I can be bummed and beaten. I can accept that I waited too long. That I held myself back, and now I've lost out.

Or I can get creative. Follow my heart the rest of the distance I threw it. See what I can do.

That one, I decide. The second one.

I'm not sure how I'm going to do it, or if I'll succeed, but at least I'm going to try.

Chapter Twenty-Seven

Melinda's sleeping down the hall in her old bedroom.

Rachel's in bed next to me. "I've had one glass of wine too many to drive home," she announced, after her fourth egg roll. "I'm staying here tonight." She then reached out and poured an extra glass of wine.

I switch out the light and into the dark of the room she says. "No kicking, no snoring, and no twitching. Capiche?"

I don't answer.

"Ellie," she says. "Did you hear me? I need my beauty sleep."

"I heard you," I say. "I just ..."

"Just what?"

"I have a problem."

"Tell me," she says.

So I do. "... and the men's game is at noon, which would be tight, but would still get him back in time for the wedding, but the women are playing after, and they're all on the same bus, so ..."

Rachel's quiet for a minute, and I wonder if she's fallen asleep. "Rach?" I ask.

She stirs, and says, "So, obviously, the thing you need to do is go pick him up."

Oh, my sister. I love my sister. "I was hoping you'd say that." My grin comes through in my voice even if she can't see it in the dark.

"I suppose you were also hoping I'd tell you to use my car to pick him up?"

"Well, I mean, obviously."

"Oh, Ellie. Of course you can. You know that. I'll lend you my car – provided we stop on the way out tomorrow and you fill it up first. I'll also help you sneak away. But both those things are conditional on us getting a good night's sleep. So go to sleep Ellie."

"But, Rach ... how?"

"Have I ever let you down?"

I think about that for a long second. Then another one. Infuriated me? *Yes.* Embarrassed me? *Definitely.* Spiked my blood pressure, made me blush, forced me to bite my tongue so hard it nearly bled? *Yes, yes,* and *yes.*

Let me down?

No. She never has.

"That's what I thought," she says. "So just go to sleep, and trust me."

Turns out Rachel kicks. Rachel snores. Rachel twitches.

I'm starting to get a new idea about why my sister's relationships turn over so quickly.

But I'm feeling very forgiving toward her right about now, so the next time her arm flings across my chest, I grab it, and hold it tight against me, and close my eyes, and next thing I know it's morning.

***

Some people might not consider it morning, since it's still pitch-black, but I'm wide awake, and with Rachel's snoring ratcheting up to a new crescendo, there's no way I'm going to fall asleep again.

So, I run.

The temperature's bang on the freezing mark – puddles wear a skim of ice, unraked leaves crisp underfoot, and the view across the park is of green grass tipped with glittering, glistening frost which will be gone the minute the first rays of sun hit it.

So, I enjoy the early-morning views nobody else will get. I take advantage of the empty streets that allow me to run right down the middle, and I let the cold air seeping in around my ankles, and whooshing into my lungs, and watering my eyes, wake me up.

Because, no doubt about it, this is going to be a big, long, emotional, tiring day.

On Melinda's strict orders we're all at the venue by 9:00. We're sitting in a cozy room, around a table covered with juice, and fruit, and pastries, and coffee. "Now," she says. "The hairdresser will be here in half-an-hour, she's bringing somebody to do your nails, your dresses are laid out upstairs – she points to a narrow back staircase in the corner of the room – and the seamstress is on-site, so there's no need for anyone to leave here before the wedding."

I nudge Rachel and she nudges me back. I pass her my phone where there's a text from Terrell. **On the bus, heading to Kingston for our game. Sorry, no miracle itinerary changes. Can I come to the reception even if I miss the ceremony? Maybe if I wear my dress pants and shirt on the bus I can bribe the driver to let me off at the nearest crossroads ...**

"What do I say?" I whisper.

Rachel grabs my phone, swivels out of my grasp, thumbs in an answer and hands it back.

I read it. **Thinking of you right now in those dress pants and shirt. Actually, thinking of you out of them, too. Why don't you text me when the bus leaves? xo**

"Rachel!" I hiss.

She shrugs. "It's a good answer. Keeps him happy without saying yes or no."

I'm about to protest when Melinda fixes her eyes on me. I'm dangerously close to getting a school-teacher-like warning. And, I have to admit it, Rachel's kind of right.

**

Once she's texted my wedding date on my phone, I give up all pride and enter "Obey Rachel" mode.

When the hairdresser arrives, my sister pushes me to the front. "Here, do Ellie first. The rest of us would like to enjoy our coffee. Plus, let's face it, she doesn't have the patience for a complicated hairdo."

I sit in the chair.

When she asks the manicurist to paint my nails a colour called "Something Blue" saying "I want to see how it looks so I can decide if I want it," I scrunch my nose at her while spreading my hands on the table.

Sasha's mom drops her off at 11:30 so she can try on her flower-girl dress and have her hair done. "Should I come back and take her home for a while before the ceremony?" her mom asks.

"No," Rachel says. "Ellie and I are supposed to tie ribbons on all the chairs. Sasha can have lunch with us then help us do that and a bunch of other things." She turns to Sasha. "If that's cool with you?"

Sasha's eyes go wide. "Lunch? Here?"

Rachel nods. "Little sandwiches with the crusts cut off. And lemonade to drink."

Sasha says, "Oh, yes, please!" and Rachel says, "Fine, but first you and Ellie have to go try your dresses on one last time so we can make sure they fit just the way they should."

"We look like princesses!" Sasha breathes.

I smile. "Very true." Of course, to my eyes, the head-to-toe high-sheen fabric with the flouncy skirt and puffy sleeves looks very different on a twelve-year-old than on a university student, but if there's one thing I should have learned, it's to look at myself less critically and accept compliments.

I bite my tongue and add, "Thank you," and I take a picture of the two of us in the mirror, just as Rachel comes in.

"Lovely!" she says. "That fits you perfectly, Sasha! Now, you're going to change back into your regular clothes so you don't drop any lunch on that dress, then you and I have over a hundred ribbons to tie."

"What about Ellie?" Sasha asks.

"Ellie has a very important job to do, that absolutely has to get done before the wedding ..." Rachel presses a set of car keys into my hand. "... so she's going to go do that while we get to the sandwiches before anyone else can choose any."

My heart rate zooms into a new gear, and my mouth goes dry. "Now?" I ask.

"Now." She looks me straight in the eye. "I have everything under control. Go."

I give my sister a quick hug, hike up my slippery skirt, say, "Enjoy those sandwiches!" to Sasha and I leave the room.

"Go out the back door!" Rachel calls. "I can't be responsible if Melinda sees you!"

Chapter
Twenty-Eight

Melinda doesn't catch me. Rachel's car starts. My silly wedding shoes are surprisingly easy to use on the pedals. I don't get stuck behind any tractors, and I make sure not to speed too much – especially when I pass the police detachment – and it only takes me two complete circles around the block to find a parking spot near the university Phys Ed Centre.

I beep the car locked behind me, and I'm checking the time on my phone, and doing mental math, wondering how close the game will be to the end. Having a little panic hiccup when I think, *What if it started early*, and *what if it's over, and the team's gone somewhere for lunch, and I can't find him, and we're late getting back, and we miss the ceremony?*

It's probably just as well I'm so deep in my own thoughts, because I'm only slightly, vaguely aware of people staring at me as I walk through the double doors, and I hardly notice the raised eyebrows of the guy behind the big desk when I ask, "Could you please tell me which gym the basketball game is in?"

In fact, it's only when I pull open the gym doors, and step in to see the teams lined up shaking hands, and somebody points, and then somebody else, that I remember, *Oh yeah, I'm a full-grown woman dressed like a Disney princess, wearing high-heeled shoes,* and I don't have to time to be swallowed by mortification, because instead I'm swallowed by a massive hug from a tall guy who's bounded off the court, and is saying, "Ellie! Oh my God, Ellie. What are you doing here?"

"I came to get you," I say. "I hope that's OK."

"Yes," he says. "Great. I have my bag. Let's go."

***

"I'm not looking," I say.

Terrell's in the backseat changing from his uniform to his dress clothes. Rachel's car is small. And there was already a sleeping bag and pillow in the back – not even asking why – before a six-foot-six guy and his sizable duffel bag got in there as well.

There are muffled grunts, and occasional bangs on the back of my seat – an elbow? A knee? – and, when I do glance in the rear-view mirror, there's quite a bit of skin.

"OK, I'm looking a little bit, but I'm really trying not to," I admit.

He laughs. "After that text this morning I'd expect nothing less."

"Ah yes, about that text ..."

He pauses and his big brown eyes lock on mine in the rear-view mirror. "What about it?"

I swallow and shrug. "I mean, it pretty much just said exactly how I feel."

He grins. "Awesome!"

* * *

My phone starts pinging as we turn off the highway on the final approach to the venue.

I pass it back to Terrell who, sadly, discovered his legs were far too long to let him climb into the front seat beside me. "Can you please read the messages to me?"

"They're from Rachel." He lifts an eyebrow.

"My sister. This is her car. She's the reason I was able to pick you up."

"I like Rachel."

"Yeah. Me, too. Most days. So, what does she say?"

"Um, OK. Message one: 'No need to be alarmed, but Melinda has just now wondered out loud where you are. Told her you were in the bathroom.'"

I nod. "Yup. That's a Rachel answer."

"Message two: 'Melinda asking if you're still in the bathroom – how can you still be there? I said you

smuggled in your own lentil salad for lunch and it isn't
sitting well – that you need some time.'"

I sigh. "Yes. If you're going to spend time with Rachel
you must be prepared to surrender your dignity."

Terrell laughs. "Message three: 'Melinda threatening
to go into bathroom and get you, lentils or no lentils ...'"
He goes quiet.

I flick the indicator. Turn onto the driveway. "What?"
I ask.

"Nothing." He reaches the phone through the gap and
places it on the front seat.

I glide the car into the exact parking spot I took it from
just before noon, and pick up the phone. Find the rest of
Rachel's message. **You'd better really like this guy, Ellie.**

I turn right around in my seat, lock eyes with Terrell –
no rear-view mirror in the way – and say, "I do. I really,
really do."

***

"I do," Melinda says, and my tears catch me by surprise. I don't think of myself as emotional – at least not
about things like this – but she's the first of my sisters to
get married, and Bill looks so unreservedly happy, and all
the changes I've been through over the last few weeks and
months must be catching up with me, and lots of other
people are crying too.

Rachel nudges me in the ribs. "I know. No more wedding planning. We can take these dresses to the consignment store. It makes me want to cry, too ..."

Sasha's truly earned her trip to the candy bar. During the ceremony not a single flower girl or page boy wandered out of the aisle, or fell over, and nobody tripped the bride. She mostly smiled, but at one point I did hear a little growl, "Git over," she warned a straying boy, and he zipped right back into place just like the ponies at the barn.

Melinda makes us all traipse outside for photographs. My sisters' lips quickly go blue, and the thirty-kilometre-per-hour gusts of wind blow our hair straight across our faces, so she finally agrees we can take them in the bright, high-ceilinged foyer.

Terrell stands to the side and because he's there, making faces at me, intercepting small members of the bridal party when they hurtle out of place, and confusing my sister, "Who is that?" Melinda hisses as we swap positions for a new set of photos, I'm relaxed. I'm smiling without my face hurting. I'm not even worried about how I'm going to look.

I might, just, get a decent set of photos of myself out of this wedding. I hope it'll make up for my mom not having any grad photos of me.

Photos done, the festivities can begin.

Here's what I'll say about my sister's fanatical planning and rigorous attention-to-detail – they've resulted in a fantastic wedding.

For dinner, Terrell is at the "significant others" table right next to the head table where my sisters and I are on display in our dresses that make us not-quite-as-pretty as Melinda. Paige's fiancé, Nathan, is sitting next to Terrell, staring up at him with a look approaching adoration.

Turns out Nathan is a huge basketball fan, played all through high school, but wasn't good enough to go any further. "Am I really, truly, seriously sitting next to one of the best university ball players in the country?" he asks. Terrell shrugs, but I nod. "You are."

"Man, I love this family!" he says.

Sasha sits next to me at the head table. "What do you think?" I ask her.

She has traces of cotton candy around her mouth, one of the temporary **XO** tattoos provided for all the kids on the back of her hand, and a tall, frosted Shirley Temple garnished with three maraschino cherries in front of her. "I'm going to be a wedding planner when I grow up," she says. "This is way more fun than horse shows."

The speeches are not-too-long and not-too-short, and just the right mix of funny and touching.

The band plays jump-up-and-move music, and Melinda and Bill lead the dancing off with a smooth fox-trot. Once Paige and Nathan head onto the dance floor, Terrell and I follow suit.

My mom's staring and, even if it's been fun to confuse Melinda, my mother deserves an explanation. Note to self: talk to Mom as soon as song is over.

"Everyone's looking at you," I whisper to Terrell.

"No, I think they're all looking at you," he says.

For the first time I can remember, it doesn't bother me to be looked at. In fact, I'm proud to be here, with Terrell. What does Rachel always say? *Take a picture; it'll last longer* ... yeah, go ahead.

When the song's over, Nathan grabs Terrell – "Let me buy you a drink" – and I go see my mom.

We stand and watch as Sasha dances with each of the guests under ten years old; taking them onto her feet and twirling them around.

"She's a lovely girl," my mom says.

"She is." I agree.

My mom turns to me. "You brought someone else who seems lovely."

"He is, Mom. I'm sorry it was all last-minute ... it just was. I promise I'll introduce you."

She smiles. "If you can, great, but just enjoy your evening. I have a feeling I'll have a while to get to know him."

I laugh. "I hope so." Then I point, "Look!" Sasha's moved onto dancing with the grown-ups – my dad is currently whirling her around the dance floor.

Sasha has dances with Nathan, Bill, and Terrell. Finally, when I'm watching her being whirled around the dance floor by Rachel's current flame, Rachel comes and stands next to me.

"She'd better not steal my guy. I've pre-paid our hotel room tonight and I want my money's worth."

"I wouldn't worry. You're really rocking the ugly dress." Somehow Rachel's pulled it off – I'm pretty sure she's had something about the dress altered – it looks a million times sexier than at our fitting, and the slight under-eye smudge of her make-up, along with the fact that she's barefoot with her high heels dangling from one hand, make her look very much like a girl who'd be fun to spend the night in a hotel with. "She is charming though, isn't she?" I ask, as Sasha spins by us.

"She is, but she's not the one I'm interested in." Rachel juts her chin toward the bar where Nathan's talking to Terrell again. "Are you happy?"

"So happy. I owe you."

"Anytime, Sis. Believe it or not, I really didn't want to have to take those boots away from you."

When Melinda throws her bouquet, Terrell lifts Sasha high over his head and she nabs it out of the air. While she's still up there, she yells, "Best wedding ever!" and Melinda answers, "Best flower girl ever!" and it's a great high note for a very tired Sasha to go out on.

**

Terrell and I walk Sasha to the front door, where her mother's waiting to take her home. We wave as the car trundles out along the driveway, then turn back into the warmth of the building.

Except.

"Not that way," I shake my head as Terrell automatically heads back to the main room.

"Oh no? Where then?"

"Not far. Just here." I lead him into the side room, where the hair dresser set up this morning. It's dark and warm. Most importantly, it's quiet and empty. I step up onto the first step of the narrow back staircase. "Perfect."

"What do you mean?" he asks.

I put my hand on the top of my head, move it across to his. "Now we're the same height."

"Is that important?" he asks.

"It helps me do this." I slide my hands along his cheeks, find the soft skin behind his ears, and brush the edges of his close-shaved hair with my fingertips.

His eyes are looking straight into mine. The rhythm of his breathing matches mine. His lips are just slightly parted, and seeing that injects me with excitement, desire, and just enough boldness to make me take one deep breath, lean in, take his bottom lip between my teeth and give it a gentle tug.

Whoa ... I'm not sure if he says it, or I think it, but I'm definitely thinking it when he responds by pushing forward and putting his lips right on mine – and they are really, really soft – and we're kissing so close our noses smush together, and our eyelashes tickle one another.

We kiss, and we kiss, and I run my hands up the sides of his dress shirt which survived the trip, and the changing in the car, surprisingly unwrinkled. My fingers ripple over his ribs, and the muscle underneath. "Sorry," I gasp. "I'm wrinkling your shirt."

"That's OK ..." Now he nibbles my lip. "I know how to iron."

"In that case, why don't you try to wrinkle my dress?"

He laughs and runs his hands over my waist, around to the small of my back. "I don't think this fabric wrinkles."

I lift my face, let him kiss my neck. "Try harder."

He takes a step up, pushing closer to me, but making it much harder for me to reach his lips. "No fair," I say, and step up onto the next tread.

We keep moving that way, *kiss-step-kiss-step*, until we've nearly climbed the stairs. His hands find the top of the low scooping neckline at the back of my dress and he slides his fingers under the fabric, spreading them wide and warm across my skin. I shiver, and overbalance, and with no more steps behind me, I tumble back and he says, "Ellie! Are you OK?"

I reach forward, and take hold of both his pockets, and tug, and he falls beside me and I say, "Yeah, fine now, thanks."

Then we're kissing on the floor at the top of the stairs. "Do you know what I'm thinking?" I ask.

"I couldn't begin to imagine."

"I'm thinking, I'm glad I went to that basketball game with Lucas."

Terrell nibbles my earlobe. "We owe Lucas."

I push myself against him as a shiver runs through me. "And I'm glad Sasha called me to help her with Oreo."

Terrell moves to my other ear. "Sasha and Oreo are a great pair."

"And ... *oooh, that's nice* ..." He repeats a series of kisses trailing up my neck. "And Rachel ..."

"We'll buy Rachel a bottle of Champagne."

I concentrate on kissing him some more and enjoying the warmth and weight of his body pushed against me.

"Do you know what I'm thinking?" he asks.

"What?"

"I'm thinking somebody's opening one of those guest room doors."

I go still and, sure enough, there are muffled voices and the rattle of a door knob. We scoot into the darkness of the back staircase and listen as footsteps head down the hall.

"Time to go back?" he asks.

"Probably," I say. "It's just ..."

"What?"

"I'm hoping I didn't wrinkle your shirt too much."

He laughs and plants a kiss on my cheek. "Funny, 'cause I'm kind of hoping you might wrinkle it more, later, just to make sure it's really worth ironing."

Chapter
Twenty-Nine

After the wedding things are the same, and they're different.

It's true my oldest sister is married, but with a date set for Paige and Nathan's wedding, I guess our family's still in wedding planning mode.

My weekdays are still filled with classes, and homework, but now I stay after school to watch Terrell practice.

I've always loved gyms – loved how such a huge space can feel cozy – it's something to do with the warmth of the wood and the height of the ceilings. I love how you need to leave the outside world behind; take off your outdoor shoes, come here prepared to work hard, or to celebrate others working hard.

Sometimes Terrell practices in the new gym – all flooding daylight and light wood. Sometimes he's in the old one – buried in the centre of the original part of the building, the floor dark with decades of use and varnish.

Either way, I take a seat and decompress from commuting, and classes, and the bustle of the day.

Often, I'll start by working on an assignment – the rhythm of the ball somehow speeding my work – or sometimes I convince Addy to come along.

To everyone else Addy might seem just the same, but to me she's a little calmer. Overall she's hopeful, but she'll also tell me when she's having a bad day. I appreciate her honesty. I'm starting to realize Addy's bubbly, out-there, try-and-do-anything personality was just the flip side of my hesitant, hold-back, caution. We were both trying to protect ourselves; just in opposite ways.

One day I look up from a Shakespeare sonnet at the sound of Rachel's heel click-clacking to the bleachers beside me. She shouldn't really be wearing heels in here. I bite my tongue and say, "Hey, what's up?" instead.

"We have a big potential donor visiting campus tomorrow. Feeling is he's going to want to direct his gift toward athletics. I thought I should actually, you know, come to the centre and see what facilities we have before I have to tour him around ... is he always that good?"

I follow her gaze to where Terrell's sinking free throws. With beautiful regularity and precision. "Um, yeah, pretty much. He's going to miss this one, though ..."

He does, and she tilts her head. "Can you always do that?"

"I'm getting better at it."

"Show me."

She watches while I say "yes" or "no" as soon as Terrell releases the ball. He sinks eight of the ten. I only call one wrong.

"How can you tell?" Rachel asks.

I shrug. "It's hard to dissect. It's the way his body moves. The way he looks. It's a feeling I get." I pause. "Yes." The ball swishes in. "It's just from putting in the time watching, I guess."

"Hmm ..."

"Hmm ... what?"

"I feel like I should try that."

I look at my sister's pencil skirt, killer heels. "Free throws?"

"No, you potato, not basketball, putting in time."

"Did you just call me a potato?"

"I'm trying to cut down on my swearing."

"Rachel? What's up? What do you mean by putting in time, and why the sudden urge to clean up your language?"

My sister sighs, tugs her slim-fitting pencil skirt upward, tries to sit, then shakes her head. "Forget it, I give up." She holds up her fingers and starts counting off. "I'm going to stop swearing, give this skirt away, and make an effort to commit to a meaningful relationship."

"What brought that on?"

She waves her hand toward Terrell. "My competitive nature. All three of my sisters are doing it. I'm sure I can manage it as well. Plus, if I let you get married first I'll have nobody to boss around when I plan my wedding."

"Rachel! Terrell and I have only been going out for five minutes. We're not about to get married."

She lifts both hands to the sky. "With an attitude like that, I can beat you no problem. Now, I need to get back to the office so I can nail down this donor tomorrow, and after that I'll get to work on Operation-beat-Ellie-down-the-aisle."

Afterward, when Terrell's driving me home, I say, "You were nearly eighty per cent on your free throws today."

He says, "I like having you there. I like that you pay attention. It makes me practice better," and him saying that gives me another swellingly happy moment like at the barn when I wondered if it was OK for me to show up early, then I found out they were happy to have me.

***

One afternoon a few alumni players drop by. The word starts moving around the gym – "exhibition game." One of the coaches turns to the stands. "Do we have anyone who can run the clock?"

I know how.

Which is to say, I've done it in the past for Lucas and Rory's teams. When the alternative was getting a parent who knew even less than me. This is different. This would be taking a chance; sticking my neck out.

Like learning to ride.

Like committing to Terrell.

I'm one part nervous and two parts self-conscious as I half-raise my hand. "Um ... I could. I mean, if nobody else can."

Which is how I end up sitting behind the console running the nicest basketball clock I've ever seen.

The first half of the game, I'm just keeping up. Or trying to. At half time the two refs roped in from their duties – one working behind the desk at the Athletic Centre, and the other a member of the women's varsity basketball team – come over. We talk over a few technicalities and "Nice job" they say.

Which relaxes me enough to remind me why I've liked doing this work ever since I sat next to Lucas at a high school game and he showed me how to do it. It appeals to my sense of detail. It makes me appreciate the game in a totally different way. I pay attention to all the players, on both teams. I notice the game, instead of the player I know best.

The game both takes forever, and flies by, when you're running the clock, and it's hugely satisfying to do a good job. To not cause either coach to complain. For the refs not to need to come over and correct the timing.

At the final buzzer I'm almost as tired as if I'd played myself. I stand and stretch my legs and turn around to face the same team coach who asked for volunteers. "Oh, hi. Thanks for letting me do that. It was really fun."

"You did a great job," he says. "We like having a group of go-to people who know how to run the clock. It's an on-call kind of thing. We pay by the game if you think you'd be interested."

It takes me a second to realize he's not just explaining things to me – he's offering me a chance to be in the rotation. "Oh. Wow. I never thought ..." *I never thought I was that good. I always thought it was just for fun.* He doesn't need to know that. "I mean, yes. I'd love that. How do I sign up?"

"If you give me your contact info I'll add you to the list."

I'm still in a daze as I wait outside the change rooms for the lift home Terrell always gives me. He comes out, bag slung over his shoulder, walking with the easy looseness in his stride I already know so well. As soon as he sees me, he grabs my hand and pulls me along.

"What?" It's hard to keep up with him.

He doesn't let go, just strides through both sets of doors and bursts into the crisp dark cold of a night with frost already glinting off the pavement.

Instead of heading right, toward the parking lot, he veers left, around the side of the building, to a courtyard abandoned in the sub-zero temperatures. He drops his bag, takes my face between his hands, and kisses me, hard.

He's caught me on an exhale, and the adrenaline and shortness of breath send sparks exploding through me when I kiss him back.

When I finally can't put off taking a breath, I pull back and say, "What was that about?"

"You didn't tell me you could run the clock."

I blink. "I can run the clock."

"That is super-hot."

I laugh. "I'll have to thank Lucas for teaching me."

"As long as he never kissed you after."

I reach up for another kiss. "You're the only kisser for me."

***

I'm also still riding, but it's different too, because now I'm done my Learn to Ride and I'm into earning my saddle time.

I get out to the barn early on Saturday and this time I muck out all the stalls in the big barn. I guess if the novelty of mucking out stalls was going to wear off, it would be when I'm doing twelve of them. But even by the end, I really don't mind.

Sasha comes along and shows me how to sprinkle the aisles with a watering can – "to keep the dust down" – she says, and then go right down the middle sweeping a broad clean path, after which it's just a quick tidy up around the door of each stall.

Laney shows up just as I'm finished, and when she says, "Spotless!" the balloon of pride inside me is ridiculous.

"Ready to ride?" she asks.

"Definitely!"

"So, here's the thing. There are two Learn to Ride classes at the show. Walk-trot, and walk-trot-canter."

"Oh-kay ..."

"Oh! Oh-oh-oh!" Sasha's jumping up and down. She's waving her hand in the air.

"It's not school, Sash," Laney says.

"No, but she has to do walk-trot-canter. Has to, has to, has to!" Sasha runs over and grabs my arm. "You have to do canter!"

I look at Laney. "Since, apparently, I *have* to do canter, what does that mean?"

"It means you need to start today."

***

While I tack Lucas up, Sasha buzzes around. "Saying, 'You'll be great!' and 'This will be fun!' and 'Don't worry about it.'"

And, to my surprise, I'm not.

I got on this horse's back in the first place. I took him over a jump. I survived my sister's wedding. I scored a university basketball game. I kissed the best-looking guy at school. I threw my heart out in front of me, and it didn't break.

I'm going to canter.

As I lead Lucas to the sand ring I realize it might be one of the last outdoor rides I get on him. The sky is low with grey, apparently snow-laden clouds, and when I rest my hand on his neck, then pull it away, his coat is so thick the outline of my palm and fingers lingers for a second.

I'm glad we can ride indoors here, but I do prefer the outdoor sand ring, so I decide to enjoy every minute of this ride.

"Ellie ..." Sasha says from the fence.

"Yes?" I wait to be told I'm tense, my teeth are gritted, my heels are up.

Sasha shoots me a thumbs up. "You're breathing!"

I laugh. Seems like a small thing, but it's really not.

Inhale-exhale-inhale-exhale. Repeat. Forever. Lucas appreciates it. I can tell because his mouth is light at the end of my hands and he's also breathing with big, loose, snorting exhales.

Laney arrives and takes me through the stuff I already know. Sitting trot. Rising trot. Circles. Changing rein. She reminds me to keep my heels down, to keep my eyes up, but not as often as Sasha used to, and she adds in other things. Small things that would have been too much for me to even think of before but now, with my heels staying down more often, I can spare a bit of brain space to work on lifting my hands half an inch or rolling my shoulder blades back.

"OK!" Laney claps her hands. "Now for canter! Any questions or concerns?"

I give a breath so massive I can feel the lift-and-lowering of my diaphragm and say, "I'm ready. Let's do it."

"OK, circle around me."

I walk around her. She shifts, and Lucas lifts his head and cocks his inner ear toward her and pushes his body against my outside leg while his walk energy amps right up.

"What are you holding?" I ask.

"Nothing."

"Lucas doesn't think it's nothing."

"Just think of it as several feet of motivation."

"Is that a giant whip?"

"Just think of it as insurance against a trot so fast it might rattle your teeth out of your head."

"Laney ..."

"It's a lunge whip, and I'm not going to use it. He just needs to know I have it." She gives it a tiny shake and Lucas arches his neck and steps even more forward. "See? Ever heard the expression 'Speak softly and carry a big stick?'"

Maybe not quite as poetic as "Throw your heart over," but I do admire Laney for having a motivational quote for each learning point.

"Does that mean I get to speak softly?" I ask.

"Definitely – as long as you also speak clearly. I'll tell you how ..."

**

"Can-ter!"

I don't know if it's Lucas's training, or Laney's motivational lunge whip – I'm pretty sure it's not the brand-new, strange-feeling aids I'm still learning (*am I really supposed to put my outside leg back that far?*) – but there hasn't been one bit of breakneck trot.

"Prepare to canter," Laney tells me, then, "Remember your aids," (*yeah, yeah, leg jammed right the heck back*), then, "Can-ter!"

I try to time my inside-leg squeeze, and my not-gripping-with-the-reins-at-all to coincide with her singsongy, "Can-ter!" and so far, every single time, Lucas has hopped up and forward like a rockstar.

The problem is, each time Laney's almost immediately bellowed, "Trot!"

What? I thought the first time as we instantly dropped back to trot.

Seriously? I thought the second time.

"OK, hang on – we just got started!" I say the third time.

"Sorry?"

"That was like – what? A quarter of a circle of canter?"

Laney nods. "Four strides, to be exact."

"Is four strides really *cantering*?"

Laney smiles. "Here's the thing – most people aren't afraid to canter. They're afraid of not being able to stop. So, if you're telling me you're sick of stopping, then I'd say we've skipped that particular phobia."

"Laney, I am sick of stopping."

"Ellie, take that horse up to a canter and go around the entire ring."

I jam my heels down, and adjust my reins, and make sure my back is nice and straight, and I breathe, and give the canter aids, and Lucas's ears only flick to me, not to Laney and her giant – if silent – lunge whip. He springs into a canter, and after four strides his ears flick back

• 298 •

again, but I give him a little nudge, "We're going!" I tell him.

We round the corner and face the long straightaway, and his ears are forward, and this is definitely faster than a trot, but I know how to keep my heels down, and I've learned to trust this horse, so I keep quiet and somewhere in the background I can hear Sasha's voice calling, "One-two-three, one-two-three ..." and I can feel it, too, and it is just like a rocking horse.

When we've gone all the way around, Laney says, "Take him through that first corner one more time, and bring him down to a trot before "B"!

I finish my trot around the ring with wind-whipped tears streaking my cheeks and my heart hammering away, and my lungs pumping, and Laney says, "Well, you look like a walk-trot-canter competitor to me!"

Chapter Thirty

The show is perfectly perfect.

The day is unseasonably warm, partly because of the brilliant sunshine and not a lick of wind.

Which is useful because I look so crazy good in Em's show clothes – even with balled-up newspaper shoved in the toes of her tall boots, and the breeches so tight I'm afraid to breathe in them – that I really, really don't want to have to cover up in winter gear.

This place – well from the long, long, straight drive lined with mature, equally spaced maple trees which manage to look regal even with no leaves left on them, to the unbroken runs of white-painted board fence, to the general calm bustle of simultaneous classes in multiple rings – it's just incredibly beautiful.

All the horses here are impressively turned out and Lucas fits right in. He's been trace clipped, which isn't a thing I knew about, but now that his coat's so thick it's meant to let him exercise without overheating. The effect is that all the parts of him that have been clipped are an entirely new shade of chestnut, and he looks very distinguished. His mane is in a row of neat, tiny, nubs – so small I don't know how Em even did them. His tail – the tail Em normally despairs of – is contained in a tight, even braid and then flows beautifully out of it with not one single clinging shaving to mar the effect. As a finishing touch, Em clipped an impeccable heart into his rump and there it sits as a reminder to me to just go with the flow, breathe, smile, and follow my heart.

I follow it right into the ring and bring my nerves with me, but they're good nerves. The kind I used to have back in the height of my ringette career. The kind that told me I was alert, and ready, and I cared enough to give it my all.

I give it my all.

Heels down, *smile*, thumbs up, *inhale*, back straight, *exhale*, check my diagonal, *relax*.

It's fine. It's good. I start on the right rein in a walk with impulsion, just like Laney told me to, and I smile, just like Em told me to, and I listen to the judge's instructions, just like Sasha told me to ("Just pretend it's me bossing you around, and you'll be fine"). And I *am* fine. They don't ask me to do anything I can't already do. Lucas is his usual rock-solid, eager-but-not-flighty, sweet-and-willing self.

An older woman cuts me off, and I just smile as hard as I can (I can hear Em's voice yelling it at me) and take

Lucas in a big, round circle to get away from her, and that takes me right by the judge, and I make super-sure I'm smiling then.

A pony ridden by a bouncing tween kicks at Lucas, and Lucas pretends it never happened. I scratch his withers and, through my smile, whisper, "Good boy!"

We're all asked to sit the trot, and for the first few strides I'm too stiff and this is where it could all go downhill, and Lucas's ears are too tense, and that's me – my fault – and I'm far away from the judge so I risk making the audible rattling exhale Sasha taught me to, and Lucas's ears loosen, and his neck arches, and his mouth lightens and suddenly my hips can follow him, no problem.

At the end of the class I line up in the middle just like Em, and Laney, and Sasha told me to and it's only then that I have the chance to count up one side of me, then down the other to find there are twelve people in this class.

Twelve. It's more than I thought.

They're pinning to sixth so that leaves me a fifty-fifty chance of taking home a ribbon.

Or, maybe a bit better than fifty-fifty because I can't imagine the rider on the pony who tried to also kick every other horse in the ring is going to place. And the lady that cut me off, well I think maybe she normally wears glasses, because the only way to describe her steering was to factor partial blindness into the equation.

The wait seems really long, and my heart swells at how good Lucas is to stand so still for me. I look across at a section of the fence I tried not to pay special attention to during the class, and now that I can really look, that swells my heart too.

There's Laney taking the time from running between rings to watch me, and Sasha giving me a not-at-all subtle thumbs-up. There's Em, crossing her fingers. Lucas stands next to her and he's just good old Lucas – calm and smiling. Then ... I swear I hear my heart ker-thump and I know I'm not imagining it, because in front of me Lucas's horsey head lifts and he cocks an ear toward me ... next is Terrell. He stands out a mile along that fence because he's the tallest, and the most incredibly handsome, and only Terrell can wear a quarter-zip athletic top and make it look like cashmere, and because his smile is just for me. It's sweet and it's wicked and, *whoa*, I need to move on because I'm still in the show ring.

Addy's gone home for the weekend, but I touch the breast pocket of Em's show jacket and feel the penny she gave me through the fabric. "I kept a bunch after they took them out of circulation," she said. "And now I give them out as good-luck tokens to my favourite people."

My group's rounded out by Rachel with her date. The person she's beginning her march toward the wedding aisle with. And I'm both surprised, and not, that he's a guy I've already met. A guy I'm inclined to like. A guy with abundant dread locks, and plugs in his ear lobes. His sweater looks like he knit it himself, but it also looks warm, as does the matching scarf wrapped around his neck. And I suppose Birkenstocks are suitable for late-fall-nearly-winter weather if you wear wool work socks under them.

"Veggie bowl dude!" Em said when she saw him, and he smiled and said, "Actually my name's Alfred," and when I'd gotten over the shock of him not being named Leaf, or Dusk, or Marley, I'd decided Alfred was perfect.

Alfred is already calling me "li'l sis," which I quite like, but which does stir a tiny bit of dread in me, because maybe Rachel's got this guy right where she wants him, and if I thought Melinda was a bridezilla, I'm pretty sure Rachel will make her look like Pollyanna.

Finally the speakers crackle. "Now for the results of Class One-A in the Learn to Ride division of the Stonegate Autumn Spectacular Schooling Show ..."

The introduction's so long I start day-dreaming. I don't love the washy pink of the sixth-place ribbons. And the yellow and white of fourth and third seen like they'd get dirty quite easily – especially if you hung them on a horse's stall. Fifth is a nice deep green. I'd take fifth, for sure.

"... and in fifth place ..." A very cute girl with lots of freckles and a big smile rides forward. *Hmm ... it is possible her smile's better than mine. She probably deserves my fifth.*

I catch Sasha's eyes and shrug. *Oh well, it was fun anyway,* and she shakes her head. *"Wait,"* she mouths.

I come second.

"What?" I actually blurt it out loud when they say, "In second place, After Lucas, owned by Em McElvoy, ridden by Ellie Hannaman."

"Oh, yeah!" Sasha says that out loud, too.

My cheering gallery cheers, and I ride out of the ring with my beautiful bright blue ribbon – which will fare just fine on Lucas's stall, thank-you-very-much – pinned to the bridle, and Sasha jumps up beside me and says, "That's what I'm talking about. Now you can win first in the next class."

***

After the show, everyone disperses. Rachel and Alfred have a potluck tonight. "I'm making lentil chili," Alfred says. "And I'm adding bacon to it," my trouble-making sister says.

Alfred wraps me in a bear hug. "Great job, li'l sis."

I make eye contact with Rachel, make a show of sniffing his shoulder, and mouth, *"No fried onions,"* and she bursts out laughing. "I know. You're right."

"Huh?" Alfred pulls away and looks between the two of us and I say, "Nothing really. She was just thinking how much she likes you."

Over Em's protests: "I should stay. Ellie could use my help. I can't just leave ..." Lucas hustles her into the car. "You can't stay. We'll miss our train. We have to go now."

"Go," I tell her. "And thanks for everything. Lucas is fine," I point to where he's blissfully oblivious to everything but the contents of his haynet, "And I'll make sure he gets put away properly back at the barn."

Sasha appears with a good-natured Oreo who is completely unfazed by the fact that two poster boards tied across his saddle declare him to be an **Oreo** cookie and that he's being led by a giant carton of milk with Sasha's arms and legs poking out of it. *Such a good pony.*

"We won the costume class!" Sasha says. "And, did you know, instead of a ribbon they gave me a five-pound bag of chocolate, and the class was sponsored by the chocolate-maker in the village, so it's, like, totally real high-quality chocolate, and that chocolate is so nice I've never had it before because my mom says we can't make the car payments, and also afford it and, also there was bag of carrots for Oreo?" She doesn't breathe once through the entire sentence.

"Sash?"

"Yes?"

"How much of that chocolate have you already eaten?"

"Good point, Ellie. I think I need to go run some laps around the showgrounds. Can you take care of Oreo?"

"I got this," Terrell says, and holds out his hands for the reins Sasha tosses in our direction as she sheds her milk-carton shell and takes off.

Oreo bumps his face against Terrell's thigh, and I say, "Aw, you two have bonded."

Terrell shakes his head. "I'm still trying to figure out this riding thing. In basketball it's two teams, playing for a set amount of time, same rules for everyone. Winning team gets a point, or a medal, or a t-shirt." He shakes his head. "Here ... costume classes. Chocolate prizes. You dressed up like ... like ... like the hottest thing I've ever seen."

I do up the buttons on Em's borrowed jacket, strike a pose. "Hot? Really?"

"I mean, yeah, in a covered-up-from-head-to-toe kind of way."

I laugh. "I get you. It's all still kind of a mystery to me. Today was literally me going where other people told me to and smiling a lot. I probably didn't understand it any more than you did. But ..."

"But what?"

I step closer to him. Pretend it's to scratch Oreo behind the ears, but I also snake my hand around his waist. "It's been good for me. It's given me confidence. I've learned lots."

"Like what?"

"Oh, there was this thing Laney told me."

"Which was?"

"Hmm ... come to think of it, it might be better to show you, than to tell you."

I lay my hand flat against his chest, until the beating of his heart pulses against my palm. "OK, now feel what your heart does when I do this ..." I stand on tiptoes and push my lips against his, and let's just say my heart isn't the only one jumping up and racing ahead.

PLEASE LEAVE A REVIEW!

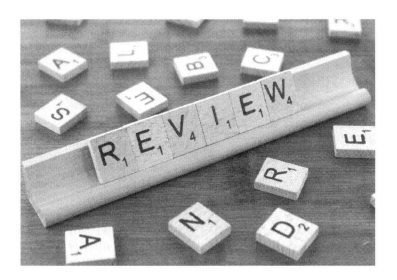

Reviews help me sell books. More sales let me write more books. A simple star rating and a few quick words are all that's needed to help other readers evaluate my books and, hopefully, buy them!

To review on **Amazon**, please follow this link – https://tinyurl.com/TudorAmazon – and select the book you want to review.

To review on **Goodreads**, this is the link – https://tinyurl.com/TudorGoodreads.

If you liked this book ...

... you might enjoy Tudor's other books. Read the first chapter of *Appaloosa Summer*, the first book in the Island Series, to find out.

Chapter One

Appaloosa Summer • Island Series
Book One

I'm staring down a line of jumps that should scare my brand-new show breeches right off me.

But it doesn't. Major and I know our jobs here. His is to read the combination, determine the perfect take-off spot, and adjust his stride accordingly. Mine is to stay out of his way and let him jump.

We hit the first jump just right. He clears it with an effortless arc, and all I have to do is go through my mental checklist. Heels down. Back straight. Follow his mouth.

"Good boy, Major." One ear flicks halfway back to acknowledge my comment, but not enough to make him lose focus. A strong, easy stride to jump two, and he's up, working for both of us, holding me perfectly balanced as we fly through the air.

He lands with extra momentum; normal at the end of a long, straight line. He self-corrects, shifting his weight back over his hocks. Next will come the surge from his muscled hind end; powering us both up, and over, the final tall vertical.

It doesn't come, though. How can it not? "Come on!" I cluck, scuff my heels along his side. No response from my rock-solid jumper.

The rails are right in front of us, but I have no horse-power – nothing – under me. By the time I think of going for my stick, it's too late. We slam into several closely spaced rails topping a solid gate. Oh God. Oh no. Be ready, be ready, be ready. But how? There's no good way. There are poles everywhere, and leather tangling, and dirt. In my eyes, in my nose, in my mouth.

There's no sound from my horse. Is he as winded as me? I can't speak, or yell, or scream. Major? Is that him on my leg? Is that why it's numb? People come, kneel around me. I can't see past them. I can't sit up. My ears rush and my head spins. I'm going to throw up. "I'm going to ..."

***

I flush the toilet. Swish out my mouth. Avoid looking in the mirror. Light hurts, my reflection hurts, everything hurts at this point in the afternoon, when the headache builds to its peak.

Why me?

I've never lost anybody close to me. My grandpa died before I was born, and my widowed grandma's still going strong at ninety-four. She has an eighty-nine-year-old boyfriend. They go to the racetrack; play the slots.

If I had to predict who would die first in my life, I would never, in a million years, have guessed it would be my fit, young, strong thoroughbred.

Never.

But he did.

Thinking about it just sharpens the headache, so I press a towel against my face, blink into the soft fluffiness.

"Are you OK?" Slate's voice comes through the door. With my mom and dad at work, Slate's been the one to spend the last three days distracting me when I'm awake, and waking me up whenever I get into a sound sleep. Or that's what it feels like.

"Fine." I push the bathroom door open.

"Puke?"

I nod. Stupid move. It hurts. Whisper instead. "Yes."

"Well, that's a big improvement. Just the once today."

She follows me back to my room. She's not a pillow-plumper or quilt-smoother – I have to struggle into my rumpled bed – but it's nice to have her around. "I'm glad you're here, Slatey." I sniffle, and taste salt in the back of my throat.

I'm close to tears all the time these days. "Normal," the doctor said. Apparently, tears aren't unreasonable after suffering a knock to the head hard enough to split my helmet in two, with my horse dropping stone cold dead underneath me in the show ring. I'm still sick of crying, though. And puking, too.

"Don't be stupid, Meg; being here is heaven. My mom and Agate are going completely over the top organizing Aggie's sweet sixteen. There are party planning boards everywhere, and her dance friends are always over giggling about it too."

"Just as long as it's not about me. I don't want to owe you."

"'Course not; you're not that great of a best friend."

***

The way I know I've fallen asleep again, is that Slate is shaking me awake. Again.

"Huh?" I open one eye. Squinting. The sunlight doesn't hurt. In fact, it feels kind of nice. I open both eyes.

"Craig's here."

I struggle to get my elbows under me, and the shot of pain to my head tells me I've moved too fast.

"Craig?"

She's nodding, eyes wide.

"Like our Craig?"

"Uh-huh."

First my mom canceled her business trip scheduled for the day after the accident; now our eighty-dollar-an-hour, Level Three riding coach is at my house. "Are you sure I'm not dying, and you just haven't told me?"

"I was wondering the same thing."

"What am I wearing?" I blink at cropped yoga pants and a t-shirt I got in a 10K race pack. It doesn't really matter – I've never seen Craig when I'm not wearing breeches and boots; never seen, or even imagined him in the city – changing clothes is hardly going to make a difference.

Slate leads the way down the stairs, through the hallway and into the kitchen, where Craig's shifting from foot to foot, reading the calendar on the fridge. He must be bored if he wants the details of my dad's Open Houses, my mom's travel itinerary.

"Smoking," Slate whispers just before Craig turns to me. And, technically, she's right. His eyes are just the right shade of emerald, surrounded by lashes long enough to be appealing, while stopping short of girly. His cheekbones are high and pronounced, just like his jawbone. And his broad, tan shoulders, and the narrow hips holding up his broken-in jeans are the natural trademarks of somebody who works hard – mostly out-side – for a living.

But he's our riding coach. Craig, and our fifty-five-year-old obese vice-principal (with halitosis), are the two men in the world Slate won't flirt with. I don't flirt with him, mostly because I've never met a guy I like more than my horse. Major ...

"Hey Meg." Craig's quiet voice is a first. The gentle hug. He steps back, eyes searching my head. "Do you have a bump?"

I take a deep breath and throw my shoulders back. "Nope." Knock my knuckles on my temple. "All the dam-age is internal."

Craig's brow furrows. "Meg, you can tell me how you really feel." No I can't. Of course I can't. Even if I could explain the emptiness of losing my three-hour-a-day, seven-day-a-week companion, the guilt at "saving" him from the racetrack only to kill him in the jumper ring, and the take-it-or-leave-it feeling I have about showing again, none of that is conversation for a sunny spring-time afternoon.

Still, I can offer a bit of show and tell. "I have tonnes of bruises. And I've puked every day so far. And, this is weird but, look." I use my index finger to push my earlobe for-ward. "My earring caught on something and tore right through."

The colour drains from Craig's face, and now I think he might puke.

"Meg!" Slate pokes me in the back. "Sit down with Craig and I'll make tea."

Craig pulls something out of his pocket, places it on the table. A brass plate reading **Major**. The one from his stall door. "We have the rest of his things in the tack room. We put them all together for you."

Yeah, because you wanted to rent out the stall. I can't blame him. There's a massive waiting list to train with Craig. And my horse had the consideration to die right at the beginning of the show season. Some new boarder had her summer dream come true.

I reach out; turn the plaque around to face me. Craig's trained me too well – tears in one of his lessons result in a dismissal from the ring – so now, even with a concussion, I can't cry in front of him. Deep breath. I rub my thumb over the engraved letters M-A-J-O-R. "There was nothing that horse couldn't do."

Craig sighs. "You're right. He was one in a million. Have you thought about replacing him?"

If you liked the first chapter of Appaloosa Summer, why not read the rest of the book? Appaloosa Summer is available as an eBook or paperback on Amazon.

ABOUT THE AUTHOR

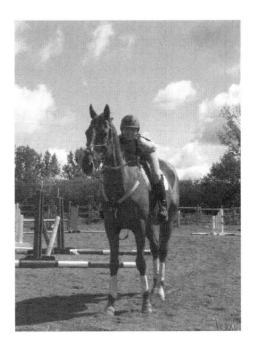

Tudor Robins is the author of books that move – she wants to move your heart, mind, and pulse with her writing. Tudor lives in Ottawa, Canada, and when she's not writing she loves horseback riding, running, being outdoors, and spending time with her family.

Tudor would love to hear from you at tudor@tudorrobins.ca .

Printed in Great Britain
by Amazon

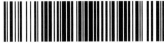